CONTENTS

CHAPTER THREE **The Routines:** *Putting It All Together*

INTRODUCTION

As you age, you're blessed with wisdom, more time to spend with family and friends, and the chance to travel. And who doesn't love those senior discounts? You do, however, have challenges. As you age, your body begins a process of gradual decline. Your bones shrink and become less dense, making them more prone to fractures. Your muscles lose strength, and your balance falters. Your memory weakens, forcing you to reach harder for thoughts that once came easily. Even your metabolism slows down. Talk about a raw deal, huh?

Are all these aging-related frustrations cause for a pity party? No! The symptoms of aging may be a fact of life, but you don't have to take them lying down. With a regular exercise regimen, you can fight osteoporosis and ward off broken bones. By working your muscles daily, you can keep them strong. If you practice balance and stability moves, you'll remain steady on your feet and recover from falls more quickly. Moving your body keeps your brain sharp and releases stress. And that pesky metabolism? Regular exercise will help it work more efficiently and will make your favorite jeans a little easier to button.

In this book, we focus on your core: the muscles, ligaments, and tendons that make up your stomach, sides, and back. We'll talk in detail about the importance of core strength in chapter 1, but we can tell you now that the highlights include proper balance, a trim waistline (critical in reducing your risk for heart disease and type 2 diabetes), and feeling good. Feeling good means being able to move around freely to play with your grandchildren, stay in your own home without assistance, drive your car, and take part in hobbies such as tennis or gardening. None of these things can happen without your health.

This book will give you the tools to move confidently through your daily life with a strong core. We will begin with a breakdown of the major core muscle groups; it's a lot easier to focus on an exercise when you know which muscles you're working and how they benefit you. Plus, we'll go over some basic do's and don'ts to help you exercise safely.

Then, in chapter 2, we'll introduce a series of 40 targeted movements broken down into four handy categories: seated exercises, standing exercises, mat exercises, and exercises with weights. We'll walk you through each movement with step-by-step instructions. In chapter 3, we'll incorporate the movements into quick sequences that will fit seamlessly into your daily routine.

You don't have to make huge changes to your life to build a stronger core and reap all the benefits that come with it. By the end of this book, you'll have the tools you need to strengthen your core muscles, maintain your balance, and retain your mobility—and they're tools you can return to again and again.

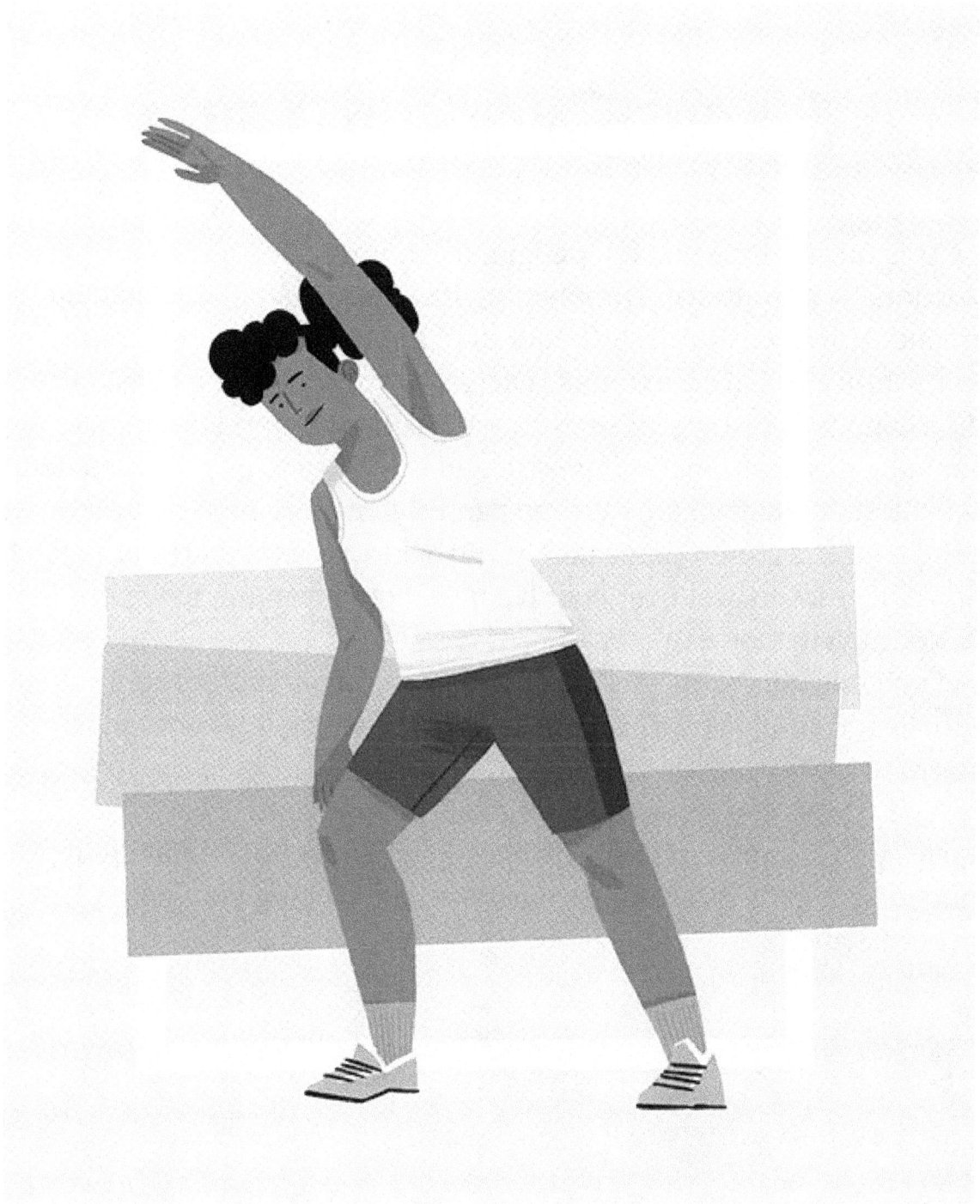

CHAPTER ONE

Your Core and You

When was the last time you felt delighted about working out your midsection? If your answer is something like *"Ha! Never,"* it would not be surprising. However, if you shift your thinking from the exercise to the effects, you'll see that core fitness is actually worth getting excited about.

In a nationwide survey of seniors, the leading aging-related concern was maintaining physical fitness. Core strength is the key to physical freedom. When you start making core exercise part of your daily routine, you'll begin to feel the effects almost immediately. You'll experience a greater range of motion and more control over your balance, not to mention feel more confident in your clothes.

As you might have guessed, core strength is about more than just being able to do 100 sit-ups. Instead, developing core strength is a systematic approach to relieving pain and preventing injuries. The core supports the spine, and if your core is weak, other major muscle groups have to compensate. This tends to throw off the alignment of your entire body, leading to pain in the back, hips, and knees, and making you more likely to lose your balance.

Learning Your Muscles

Your core is the intricate network of bones, nerves, ligaments, and tendons, along with all the muscles, that attach to the spine. These elements wrap all the way around the body, like a girdle, and even extend down below the hips.

To help you better understand the muscles of the core, we're going to get a bit anatomical. As your new core exercises become second nature, you'll think *"Aha!"* as you feel the different muscles working.

Transverse abdominis

Located on the front of your body on either side of the navel, the transverse abdominis muscles are layered below the obliques and form the innermost of the flat muscles of the abdomen. The transverse abdominis aid in breathing and are extremely important in stabilizing the lower spine and pelvis as you move.

Obliques

Your obliques extend diagonally from your ribs to your pelvis and consist of two sets of muscles: The external obliques are located directly on top of the internal obliques, with the muscle fibers in each group running perpendicular to one another. The internal and external obliques work in tandem and enable you to bend your torso sideways, rotate your torso, and round your spine. They also help brace the spine, as when you're about to lift a heavy object.

Rectus abdominis

Ah, the coveted six-pack. These highly sought-after muscles are the rectus abdominis, which run vertically along either side of your abdomen from the sternum to the pubic bone. They're what help you bend your torso forward and tilt your pelvis.

Map of Major Core Muscles

Rectus abdominis
Diaphragm
Transverse abdominis
Obliques

Erector spinae
Latissimus dorsi
Transversospinalis

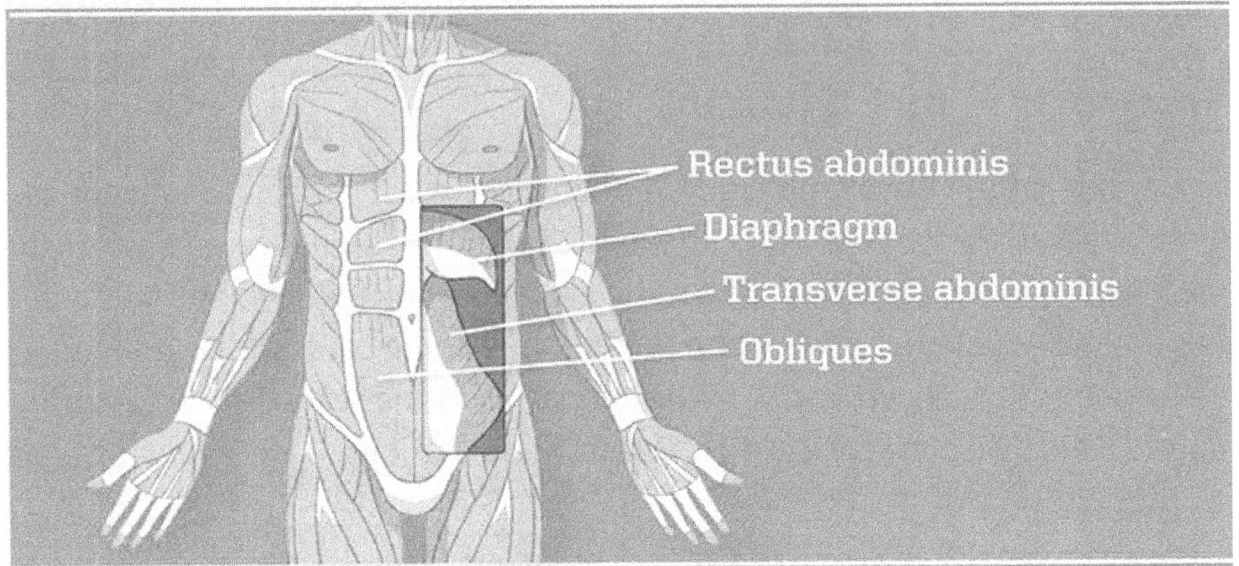

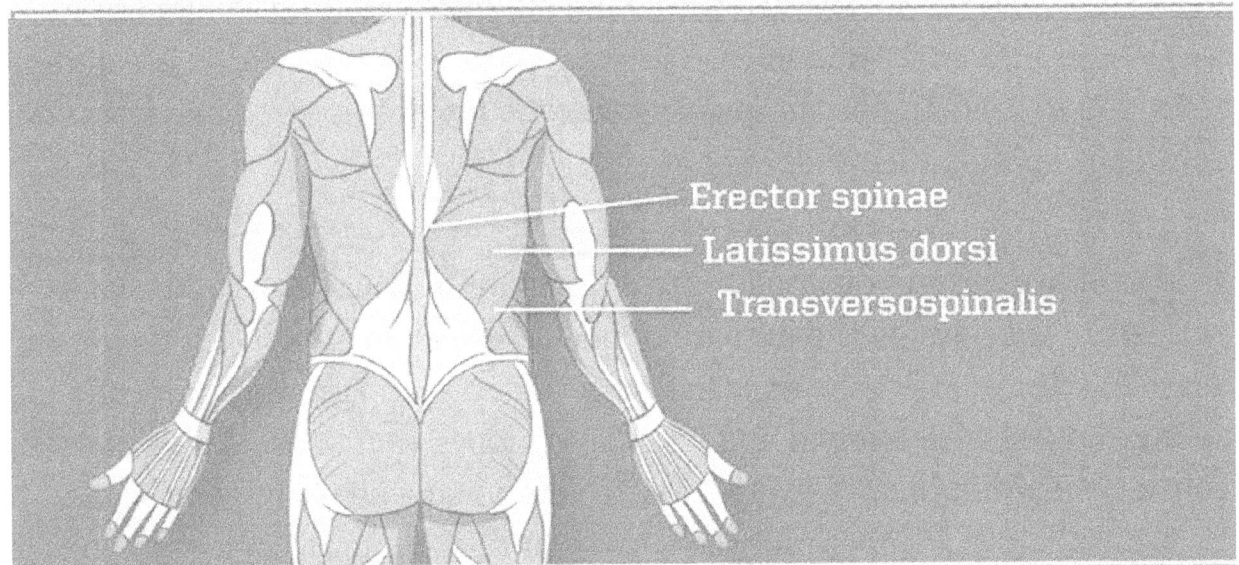

Transversospinalis and Erector spinae

These two muscle groups run along the spine all the way from the head to the pelvis. These very important muscles stabilize the vertebral column and enable spinal movement, which is critical for so many of the motions you go through in your everyday activities. The spinal muscles play a big role in proprioception, which is your awareness of the position of your body, helping keep you balanced even when you're not consciously thinking about it.

Latissimus dorsi

The latissimus dorsi (often referred as the "lats") are the largest muscles in the upper body. This muscle group runs across your back from just below your shoulder blades down to your pelvis and helps stabilize the spine and move the shoulders.

Diaphragm

Situated at the base of the chest, this muscle separates the chest from the abdomen. When you inhale, it contracts and flattens, creating a vacuum-like effect. When you exhale, the diaphragm relaxes, and the air is pushed out of your lungs. In addition to aiding breathing, a strong diaphragm helps prevent acid reflux.

The Benefits of a Strong Core

The core is key to a stable and mobile body. Let's take a look at just a few of the many science-backed benefits of strengthening your core.

Improve balance

If you have a weak core, you may feel unsteady on your feet. In fact, falls are the leading cause of injury and death for adults older than 65. Strengthening the muscles that wrap around the abdomen provides stability to the "trunk" of your body. This helps you stand steadily and move more freely.

Reduce pain

When your core muscles are weak, your posture suffers, and other muscles must make up for the lack of support. This leads to back pain, which can range from annoying to debilitating. Building core strength will help you maintain proper posture while sitting, standing, and walking, which alleviates the pressure on other muscle groups and, in turn, reduces back pain.

Stay mobile and remain independent

Golf, tennis, swimming, gardening, traveling, volunteer work . . . We could go on about all the activities that motivate you to stay mobile. The bottom line is this: Research has shown that greater mobility is linked with a higher quality of life in older adults.

Three out of four adults in your age group say they want to stay in their current home as they age, yet only 46 percent believe that doing so is a realistic possibility. Building a strong core—and in turn, greater balance and mobility—can help you safely stay in the home you love for as long as possible.

Better overall health outlook

A slimmer waistline can boost your confidence, but it also lowers your risk of chronic health conditions such as diabetes and heart disease.

Don't Forget to Stretch

If you fail to stretch your muscles regularly, they shorten and become tight. Then when you go to use them, they're unable to extend all the way, putting you at greater risk of muscle strains and tears. To reduce this risk, it's important to do some light stretching, not only before doing your daily exercises but a few times throughout the day.

Stretching also comes with other benefits besides injury prevention, many of which relate to your larger goals of staying mobile and independent in your senior years. Stretching gets your blood pumping to different areas of the body, which wards off painful inflammation. When your muscles are limber, it's easier for you to stand up straight and keep your spine in proper alignment. If you've ever felt the relief that comes with taking a big stretch after a long drive, you know firsthand the good that stretching can do for tight, tensed-up muscles.

Go slowly when stretching, and never force your body beyond what's comfortable. Proper form is more important than how far you can stretch. Many of the exercises in this book also double as effective stretches. The Metronome, Triangle, and Cat Cow exercises are a few such examples.

Don't Forget to Breathe

Practicing proper breathing while exercising keeps oxygen flowing throughout your body, allowing you to exercise more comfortably, more safely, and for longer periods. Breathing, like stretching, promotes good circulation, which is beneficial for reducing pain and inflammation.

Consistent rhythmic breathing helps prevent blood pressure spikes and painful cramping during exercise as well as reducing the incidence of hernias. Plus, focusing on your breathing is a great way to stay present with the exercise and get the most out of every movement.

If you're new to exercise or just getting back into the swing of it, controlling your breath can feel unnatural. Like exercise itself, breathing properly will get easier over time. Let's discuss a few tips to help you breathe properly through your core exercises.

Practice good posture. Standing or sitting up straight expands your chest, which allows for full, deep breaths and prevents panting.

Inhale while resting and exhale while exerting. To use a crunch as an example, this would mean you'd inhale while lying flat on your back and exhale as you crunch upward.

Don't hold your breath. Breathe in and out at a measured pace, doing your best to keep a consistent rhythm. One trick to help with this is listening to a playlist while you do the moves. Some people find it helpful to breathe in and out in time with the music.

If you can't catch your breath, slow down or take a break. Raise your arms overhead and breathe in. Lower them in front of you as you breathe out deeply, repeating until your heart rate slows. Start your exercises again when you feel comfortable or pick back up the next day.

Exercise Myths and Mistakes

Excuses for why you can't make fitness a priority come in all shapes and sizes. Some of them are the simple result of misinformation or practices that have been internalized through years of bad habits. To help you beat the excuses, let's address some of those exercise myths and mistakes proactively.

Myths

There are a few common exercise myths that many seniors buy into. Beware these exercise untruths, which can prevent you from reaching your full potential and can even lead to injuries.

I'm too old to exercise.

Tell that to one of my students, Peg, who recently turned 99 and still shows up to class regularly. Barring some very specific health conditions, exercise is a good thing for people of any age. A regular exercise routine—even one that you start after the age of 50—can significantly reduce your risk of premature death compared with someone the same age who doesn't exercise at all. If you have specific concerns about why exercise might not be appropriate for you, talk them over with your doctor before getting started.

It's too late to start.

This is, to put it plainly, a bunch of baloney. The science on this subject is actually pretty amazing. Researchers studied two groups of exercisers over the age of 60: people who'd been exercising twice a week for the last 20 years and people who didn't have a consistent workout routine. They followed the individuals within each group before and after workouts to see how proteins were developing within their muscles. Here's the amazing part: There was no difference between the two groups in the rate of muscle synthesis. So, even if you've never worked out before, you have just as much to gain from starting now than someone who's been at it for years.

I need to use weights to get a good strength workout.

Building strength is not about the weight. It's about *resistance* and making your muscles work against it. The weight of your body and limbs, combined with gravity, offers plenty of resistance to build strength. Some of the exercises in this book do call for weights, but the majority of them do not. You can even choose to modify the weighted exercises by doing them without weights.

Exercise will make my arthritis or osteoporosis worse.

Oh, how we wish this myth would go away. The reality is that *lack* of exercise is actually much worse for stiff, painful joints. Think of your arthritis or osteoporosis like a squeaky, rusty bicycle wheel. Exercising is like adding lubricant, which helps the wheel turn smoothly. The longer the bicycle—or in this case, your body—sits around without moving, the rustier it gets. Gentle movement is one of the best things you can do to ward off pain from these conditions.

Mistakes

Everyone makes mistakes, but hopefully a little forewarning will help you avoid making some of these errors.

Improper form.

Technique matters. Before you worry about building up the number of reps you can do, focus on getting your form right. Proper technique not only helps you avoid injury but also ensures you're getting the most out of the hard work you're putting into each exercise. If you have existing pain, poor technique can make it worse. We've included detailed instructions and a diagram with every exercise to help you achieve the proper positioning for each move.

Only doing cardio.

Walking every day is certainly admirable, but it's not enough to ward off the effects of aging, such as muscle loss and weakened bones. Incorporating resistance training, such as the exercises in this book, is imperative if you want to maintain the strong muscles and bones that allow you to live an independent and enjoyable life. Aim to do some type of resistance training a minimum of three times per week.

Skipping balance training.

What do you do when you want to get better at something? You practice. Believe it or not, you have to give your brain practice at being off balance if you want your body to react and catch you when you trip, slip, or fall. You can trick your brain into practicing "falling" by incorporating balance exercises into your regular routine. The Side Crunch with Leg Lift and the Diagonal Sit Back are two great exercises that will improve your balance in addition to strengthening your core.

Everybody Is Different

The moves in the following chapters are for everyone, whether you've been an avid exerciser for years or it's hard to remember the last time you set foot in a gym. The exercises are designed to be easy, accessible, and best of all, effective. Remember, take it slow. There's no need to try all 40 moves the first day. Everyone will have different thresholds for the levels of movement and exertion they feel comfortable with. Even your own thresholds can change from one day to the next. You might feel great blasting through five or six exercises today but only be up for one or two tomorrow.

It's a medical fact that your body sends up red flags to tell you when something is wrong. Feeling dizzy or lightheaded, for example, are red flags that it's time to take a break or stop. It's normal to feel mild discomfort when exercising and some soreness afterward, but if you experience sharp or persistent pain, your body is probably saying *"Stop!"*

Finally, give yourself time to rest. Although it's ideal to get some kind of movement every day, challenging workouts are not recommended seven days a week. Instead, allow yourself one to two days a week for recovery. You can still do something on these days to get your body moving, such as walking, swimming, or putting on some music and dancing, but don't push yourself to max exertion.

SEEK PROFESSIONAL ADVICE

Consult your doctor or other health-care professional before starting this (or any) exercise program. This is particularly important if you have a history of high blood pressure or heart disease; if you have ever experienced chest pain when exercising; if you smoke, have high

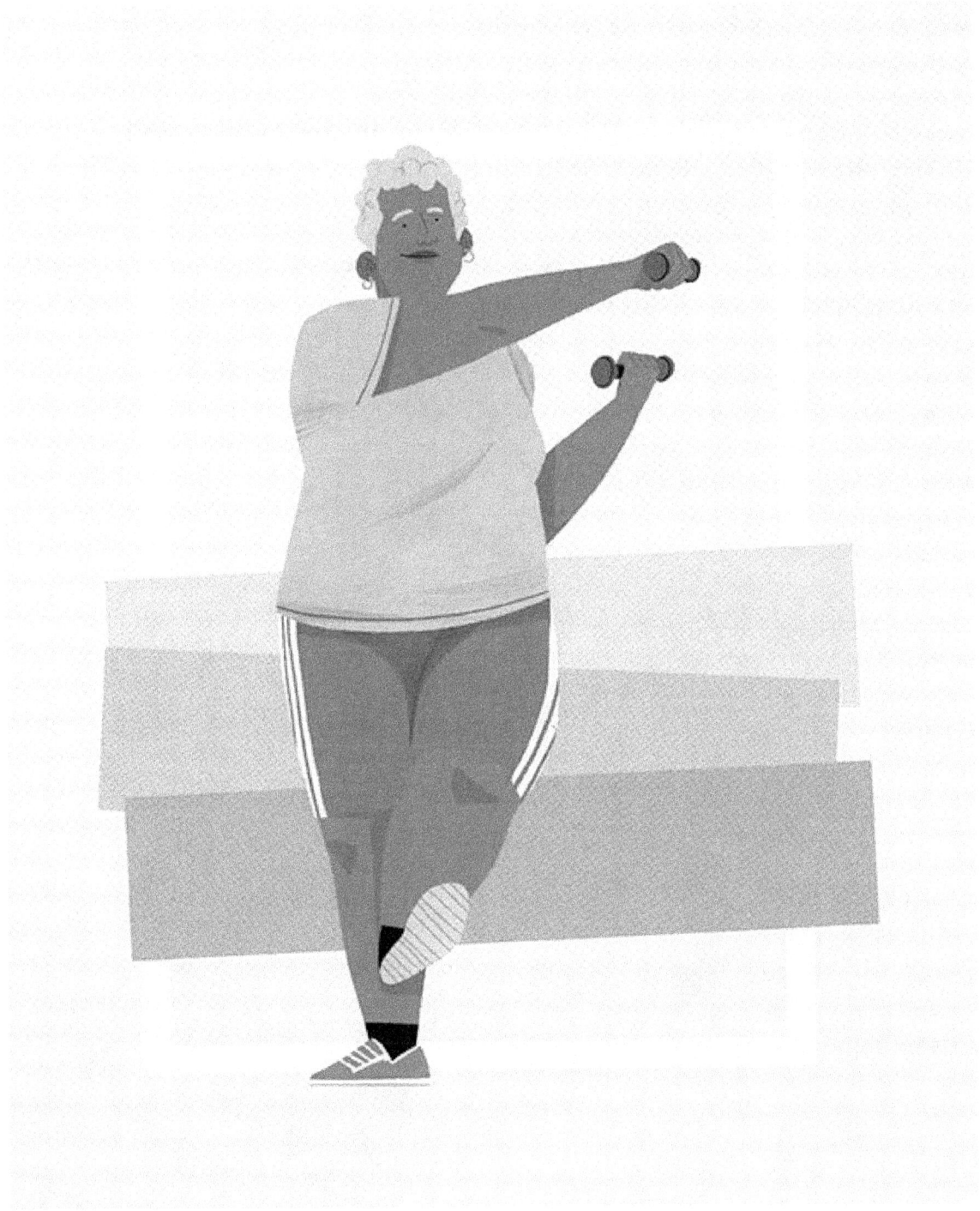

CHAPTER TWO

The Exercises
Getting Active

Now that we've laid the groundwork, it's time for the fun part: exploring your core-strengthening exercises.

This book includes 40 targeted exercises which are conveniently grouped into four categories.

Seated exercises. These are a great starting point, especially if balance is currently a challenge. Start in a chair with a nice, high back and without arms. Once you master the moves, you might feel comfortable doing these on the edge of the couch or an armchair, while watching TV.

Standing exercises. The exercises here challenge you to concentrate on your balance in addition to working your muscles, which is a great way to build muscle memory that will serve you as you move through daily life.

Mat exercises. Perform these moves on a standard yoga or exercise mat, or even on a beach towel outdoors. It's important that you protect your back, so focus on achieving proper form first, then work on reaching the target number of repetitions or length of time.

Exercises with weights. For the final ten exercises, light dumbbells work best, but soup cans or water bottles can work, too. The weight will vary for everyone. We recommend starting on the light side—two- or three-pound dumbbells are a great starting point—and increasing the weight only if you are ready for more.

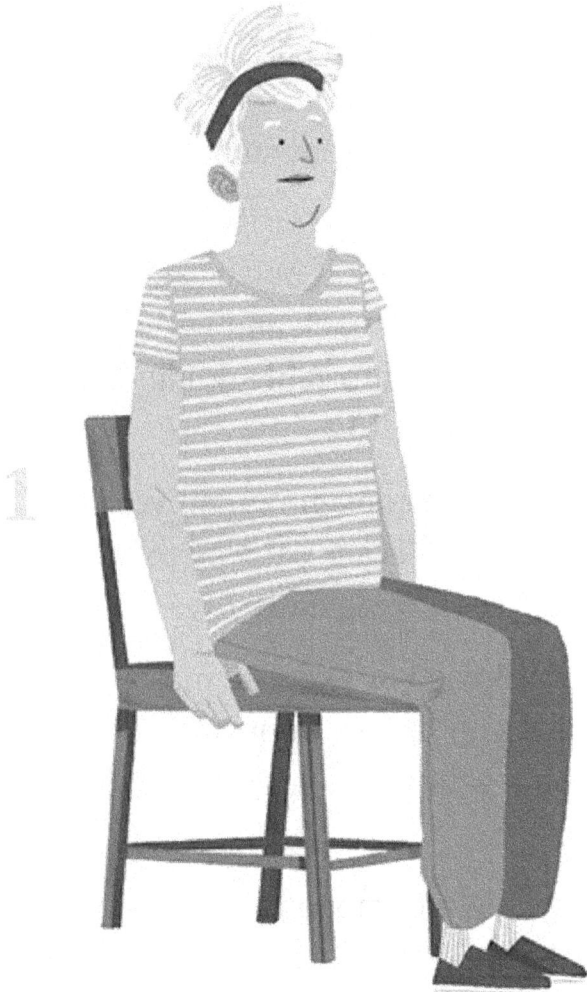

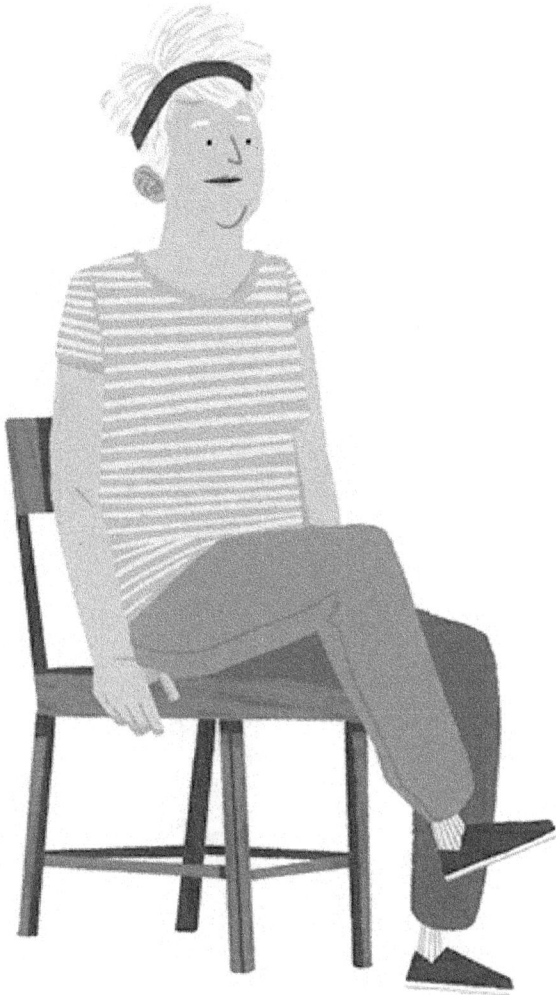

2

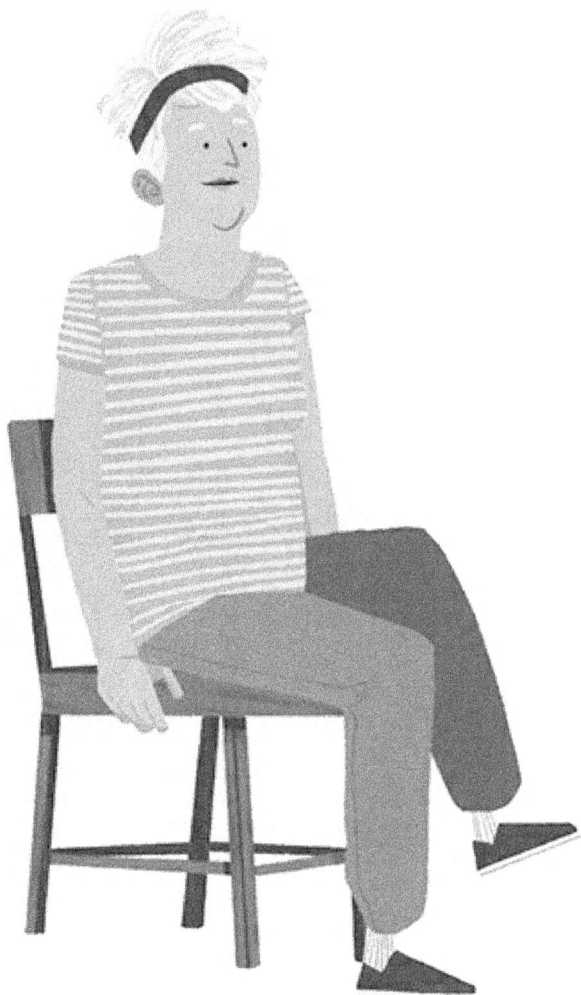

Knee Lifts

TARGET MUSCLE GROUPS

Transverse abdominis / Lower rectus abdominis

This exercise mimics the motion your lower body makes when getting out of the car. One of the worst falls I've taken happened in this very scenario. My foot didn't quite clear the opening of the car door but got stuck on the edge, and down I went. After that, I started doing this exercise more often. This move engages the lower abs while also strengthening the upper muscles of the legs, which are vital for climbing steps.

INSTRUCTIONS

1   Begin in a seated position, sitting up nice and straight. If you need to, grip the sides of the chair for stability. Inhale.

2   As you exhale, contract your abdominal muscles while raising your right leg, keeping your knee bent at a 90-degree angle. Inhale as you lower your leg.

3   Repeat on the other side. This is 1 full rep. Aim for 10 reps at the beginning and work your way up to 20 over time.

Modification: Add ankle weights to increase the resistance.

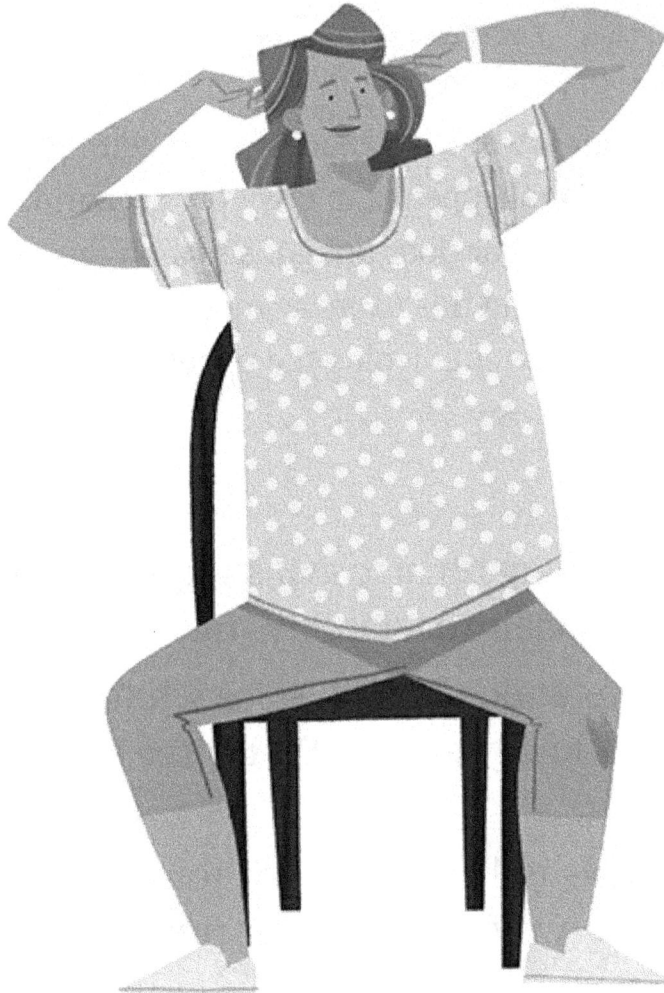

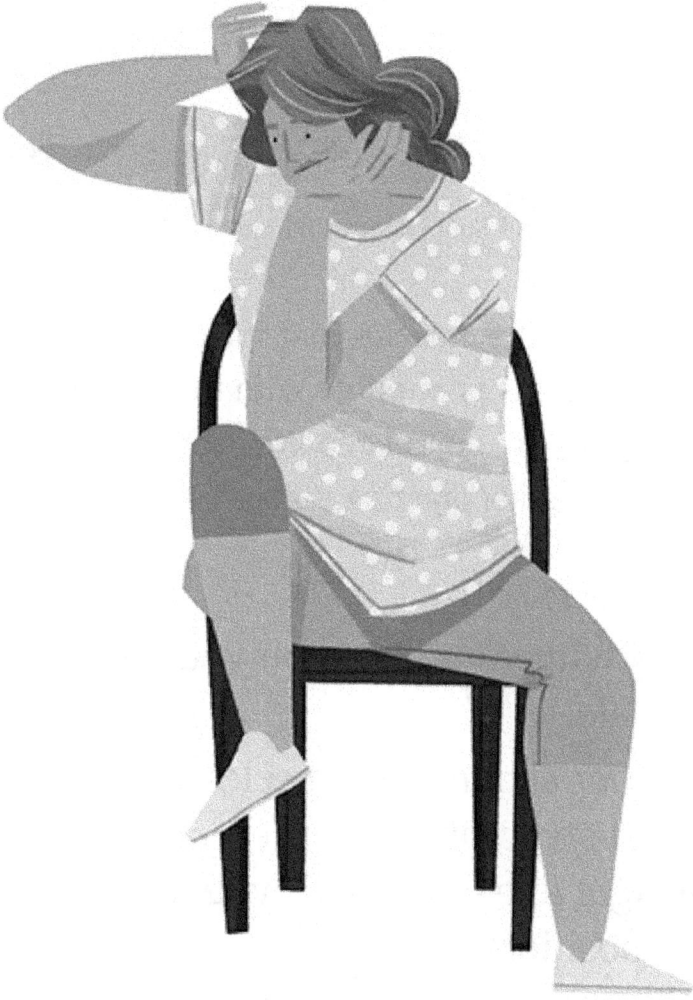

2

Diagonal Crunch

Transverse abdominis · Rectus abdominis · Obliques

This move is a low-impact way to tone the muscles that form the "six-pack" without pulling and straining your neck as is possible with traditional crunches. The seated position also forces you to keep your torso from wobbling too much, which is good balance practice.

INSTRUCTIONS

1   Begin in a seated position with your hands on your head and both feet on the floor. Inhale.

2   As you exhale, contract your abdominal muscles while raising your right leg. Simultaneously, crunch your left elbow downward toward your right knee. Inhale as you lower your leg and return to the upright position.

3   Repeat on the other side. This is 1 full rep. Aim for 10 reps at the beginning and work your way up to 20 over time.

Modification: Add ankle weights to increase the resistance.

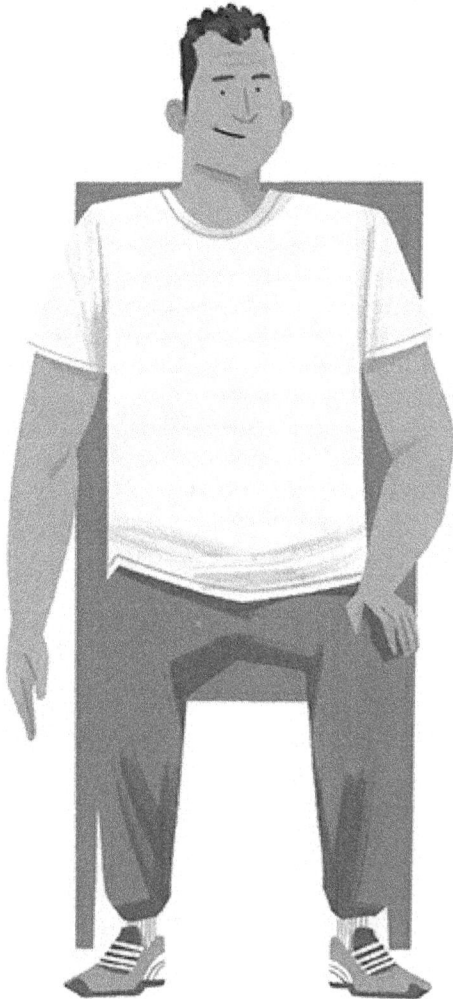

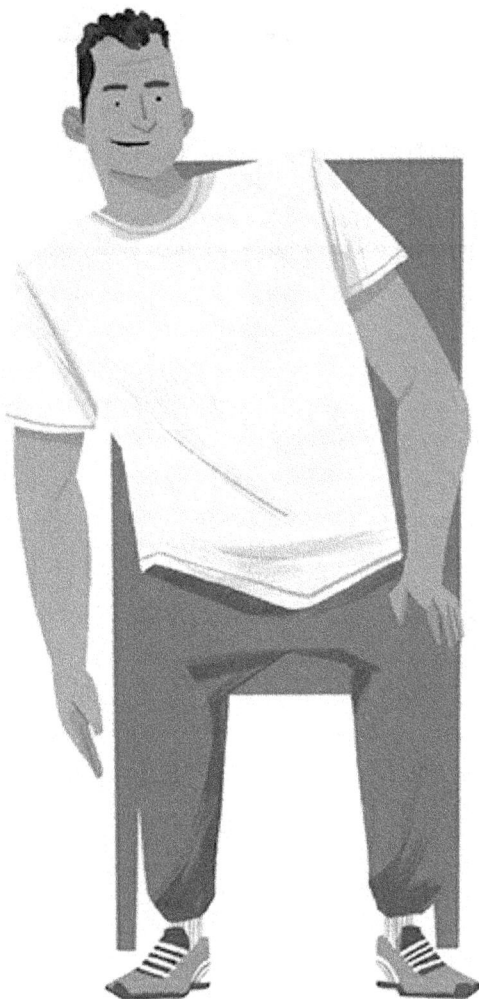

Seated Side Bend

Obliques / Erector spinae

This move works the many muscles along the spine, which you engage every time you bend over to pick up something or tie your shoes. These muscles also play an important role in proper posture, which is key for fighting off back pain.

INSTRUCTIONS

1 Begin in a seated position with your hands hanging down over the sides of the chair. Inhale.

2 As you exhale, engage your core and bend to the right, reaching your right hand down toward the floor.

3 Inhale as you return to the upright position. This is 1 rep. Repeat 8 to 10 times, then do the same on the other side.

Modification: Hold a dumbbell for added resistance.

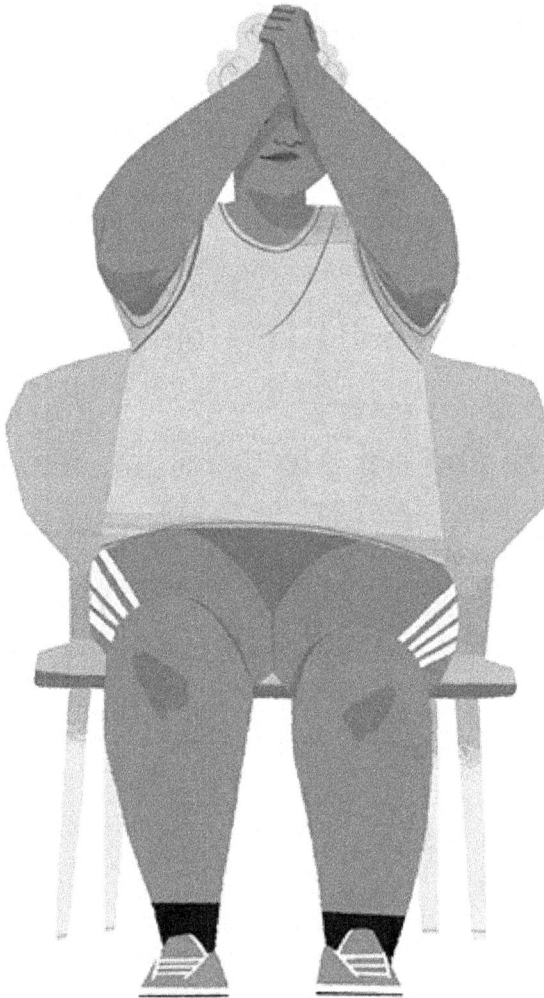

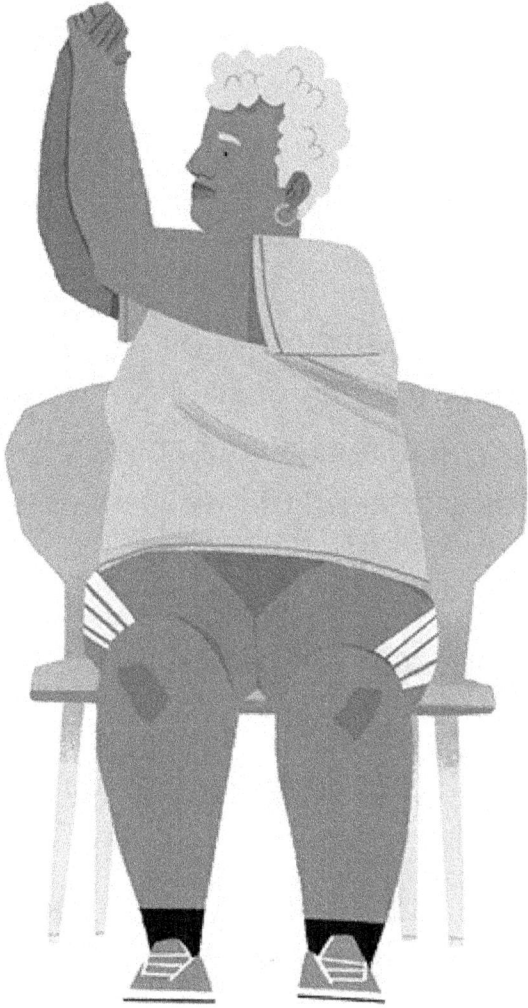

2

Seated Twist

TARGET MUSCLE GROUPS

Rectus abdominis   Transverse abdominis   Obliques

The muscles you engage in this exercise are the same ones you use when you turn to check your blind spot while driving—very important if you want to stay safe on the road. This move will help you maintain your ability to quickly change direction, plus it's great for getting rid of love handles.

INSTRUCTIONS

1   Begin in a seated position with your hands clasped, arms in front of your chest. Inhale.

2   Exhale as you twist to one side. Imagine pulling your core muscles tight around your spine, like a corset.

3   Inhale as you return to center, then exhale and twist to the other side. This is 1 rep. Aim for three sets of 8 to 10 reps.

Modification: Hold a dumbbell or medicine ball for more resistance.

Try to hold your arms level and keep your feet flat on the floor.

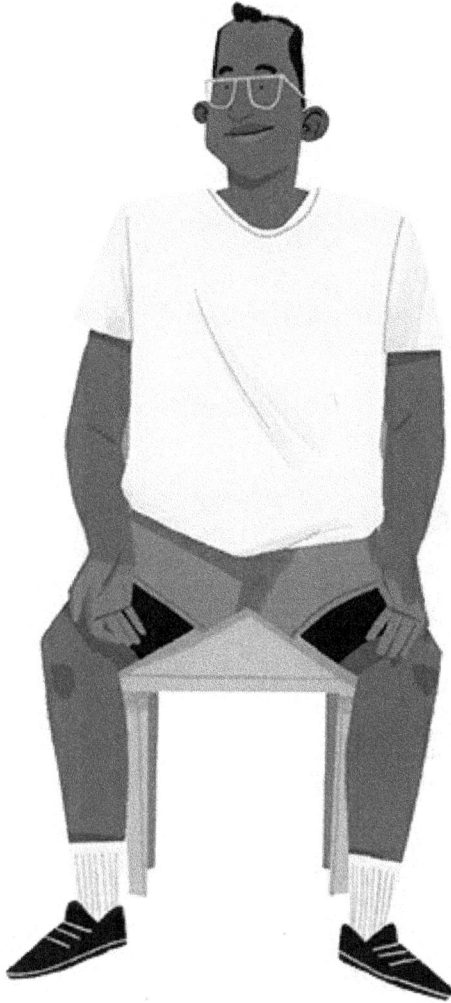

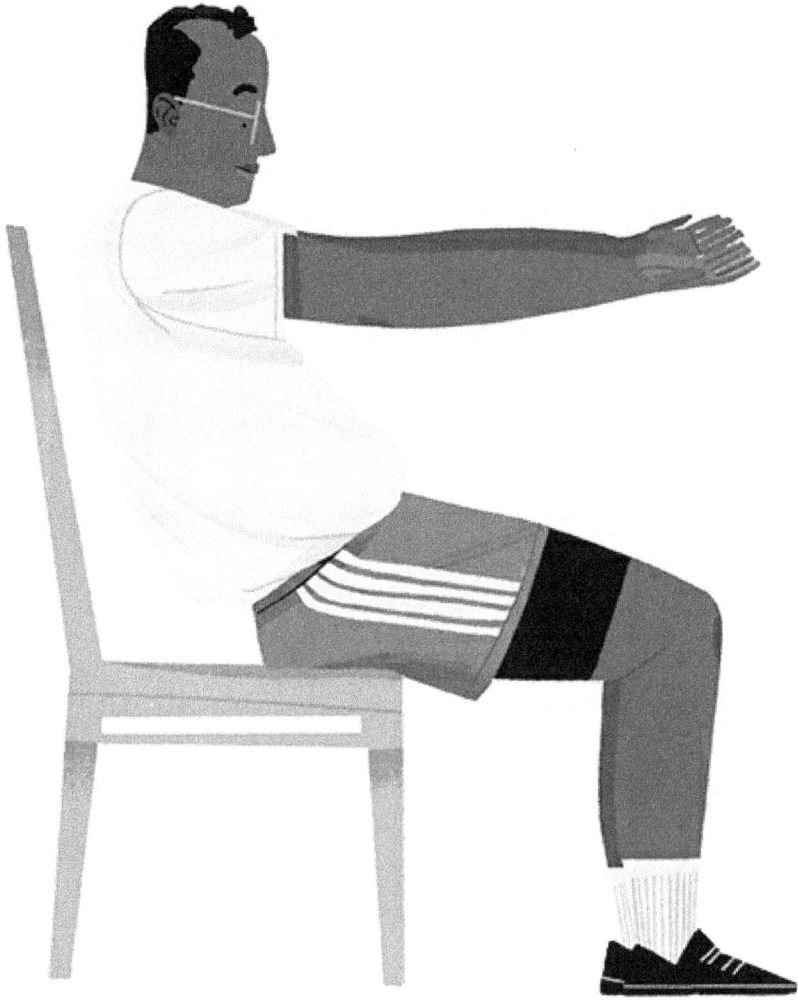

Slow Recline

Rectus abdominis   Transverse abdominis

This reclining exercise is great for strengthening the muscles you need to comfortably sit up in bed; get up from a deep, comfy sofa; or get up from the mat after a floor workout.

INSTRUCTIONS

1   Begin by sitting up straight at the edge of the chair with your arms extended in front of you, palms up. Inhale.

2   Exhale as you slowly recline toward the back of the chair, rounding your spine into a concave "C" shape. Your back may touch the chair back, but don't fully relax into the chair.

3   Inhale as you return to a fully upright position. This is 1 rep. Aim for 10 reps.

Modification: Place your hands on your hips or hold the edges of the chair to make it less challenging.

A good visual to imagine is pulling a rope across your body. Try to keep your arm elevated and parallel with the floor throughout the exercise.

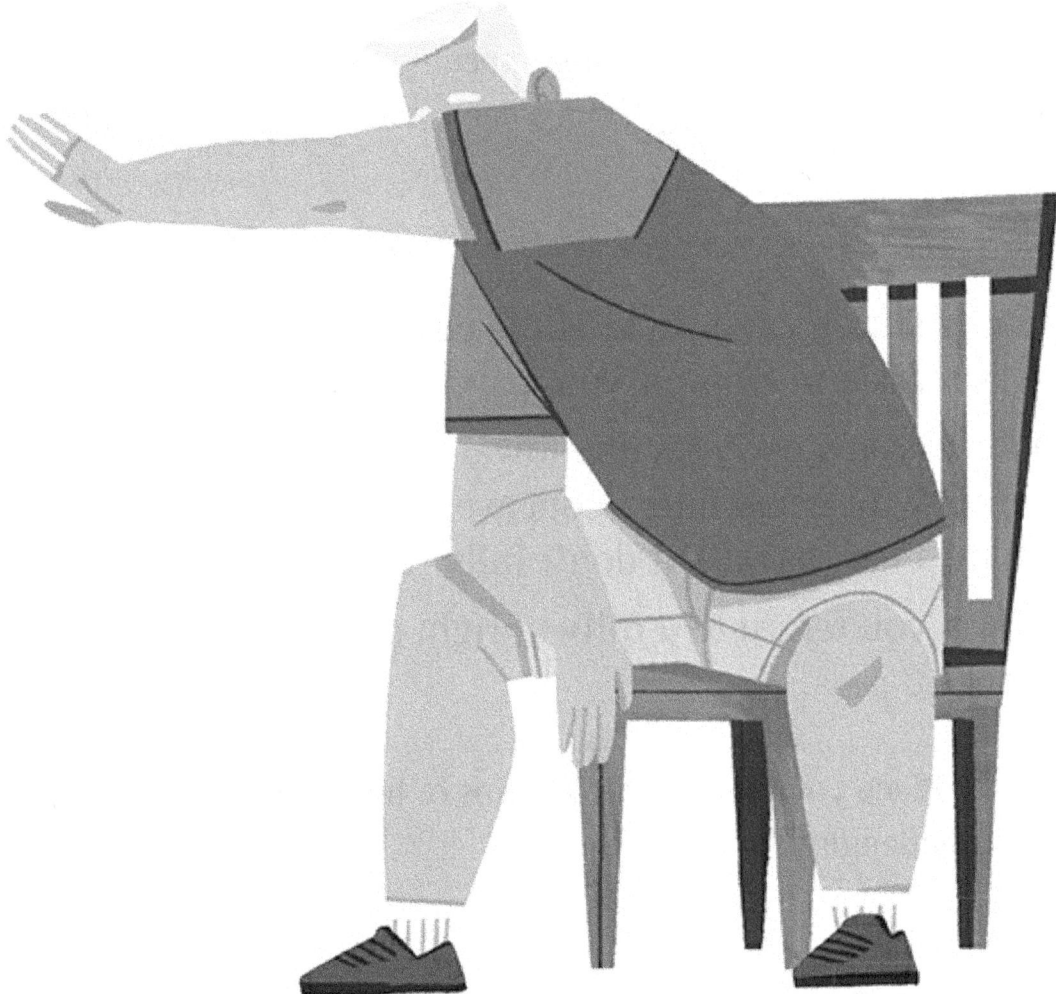

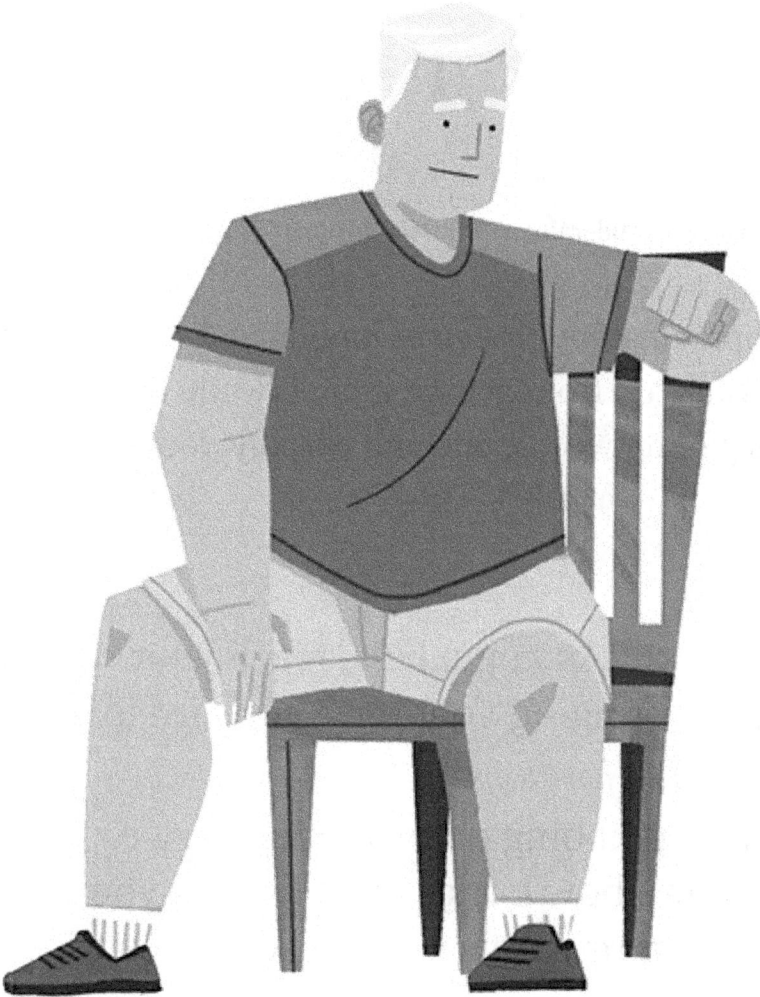

Rope Pulls

Rectus abdominis   Transverse abdominis   Latissimus dorsi   Erector spinae

This is a great move for improving your range of motion and maintaining strong lats, which help prevent you from getting injured while doing everyday activities such as pulling weeds, opening a heavy door, or unloading the dishwasher.

INSTRUCTIONS

1   Begin in a seated position. As you inhale, reach your right arm across your body while bringing your torso forward to a 45-degree angle.

2   Make a fist as if you're grabbing onto an imaginary rope. Exhale as you pull your elbow backward, bringing your fist in line with your armpit and returning your torso to an upright position.

3   This is 1 rep. Aim for 8 to 10 reps on each side.

Modification: Increase the range of motion by twisting to look over your shoulder on the pull and touching your elbow to the chair behind you.

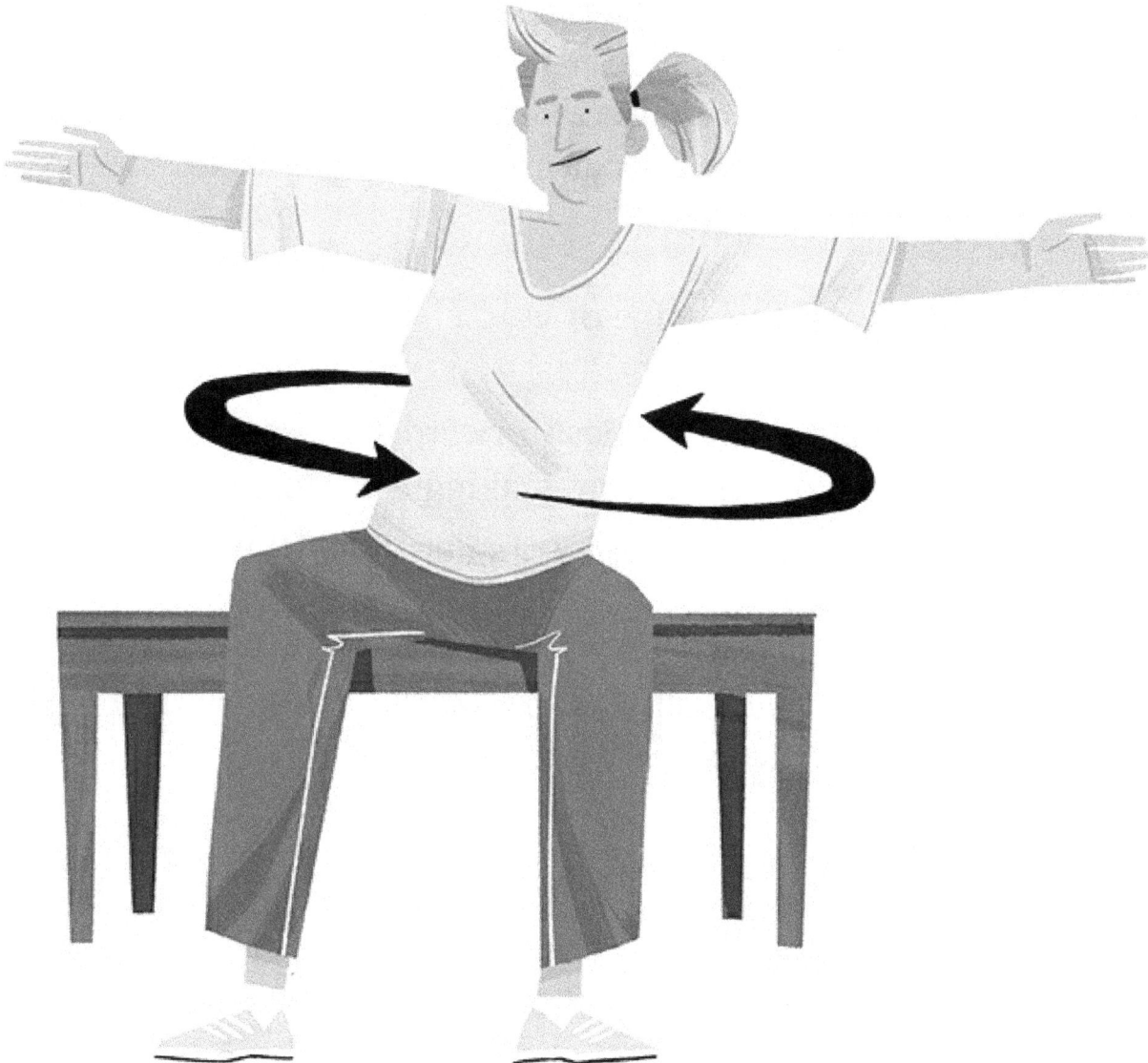

Ab Circles

Rectus abdominis / Transverse abdominis

This exercise promotes proper posture and combats the effects of sitting for long periods. Sitting for too long each day leads to muscle deterioration and all kinds of misalignment issues that can contribute to back pain. Counteract those long hours in front of the computer with this simple move.

INSTRUCTIONS

1. Sit forward toward the edge of your chair, arms outstretched to either side. Inhale.

2. As you exhale, push your chest forward and around to one side, then back in a circular motion, making a complete circle.

3. Maintain steady breath as you complete 8 to 10 full circles. Repeat on the other side.

Modification: For more of a challenge, hold weights in your outstretched hands, palms up, or hold weights and cross your arms on your chest.

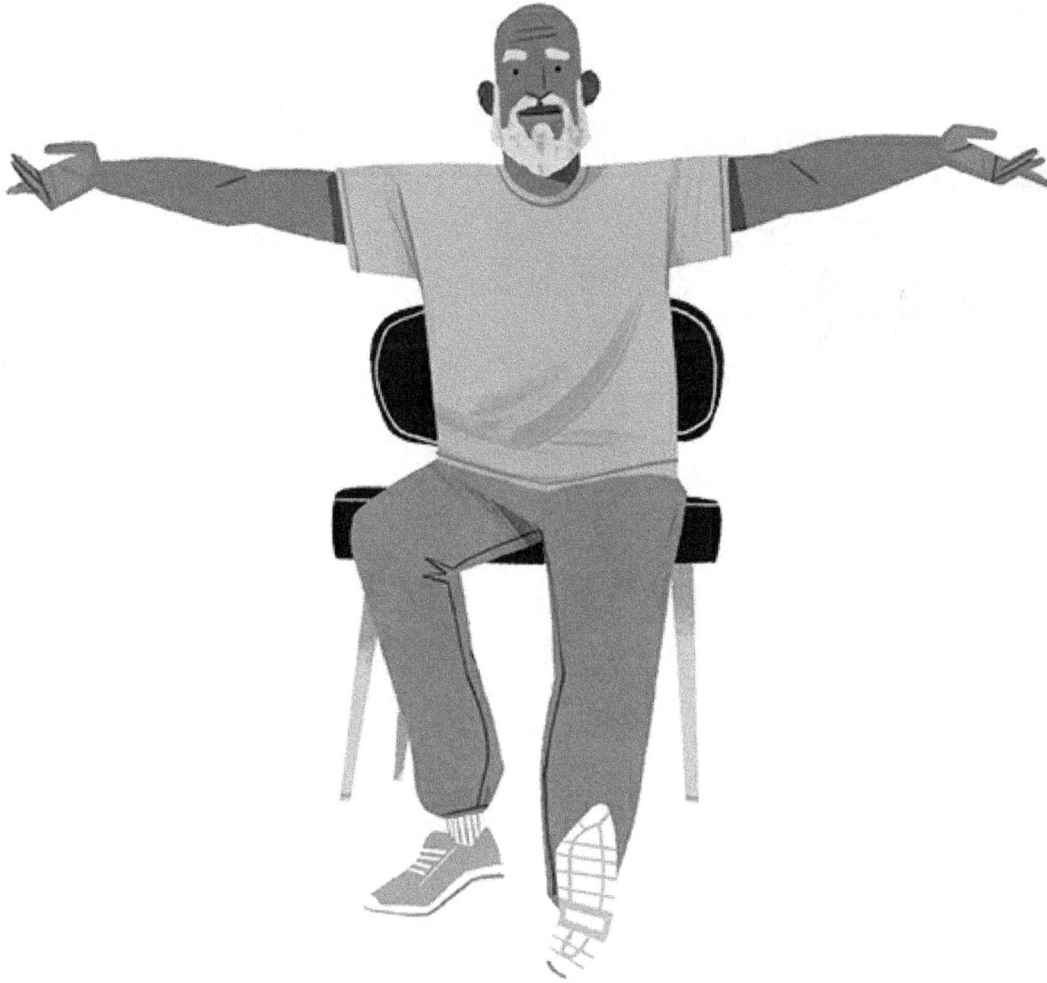

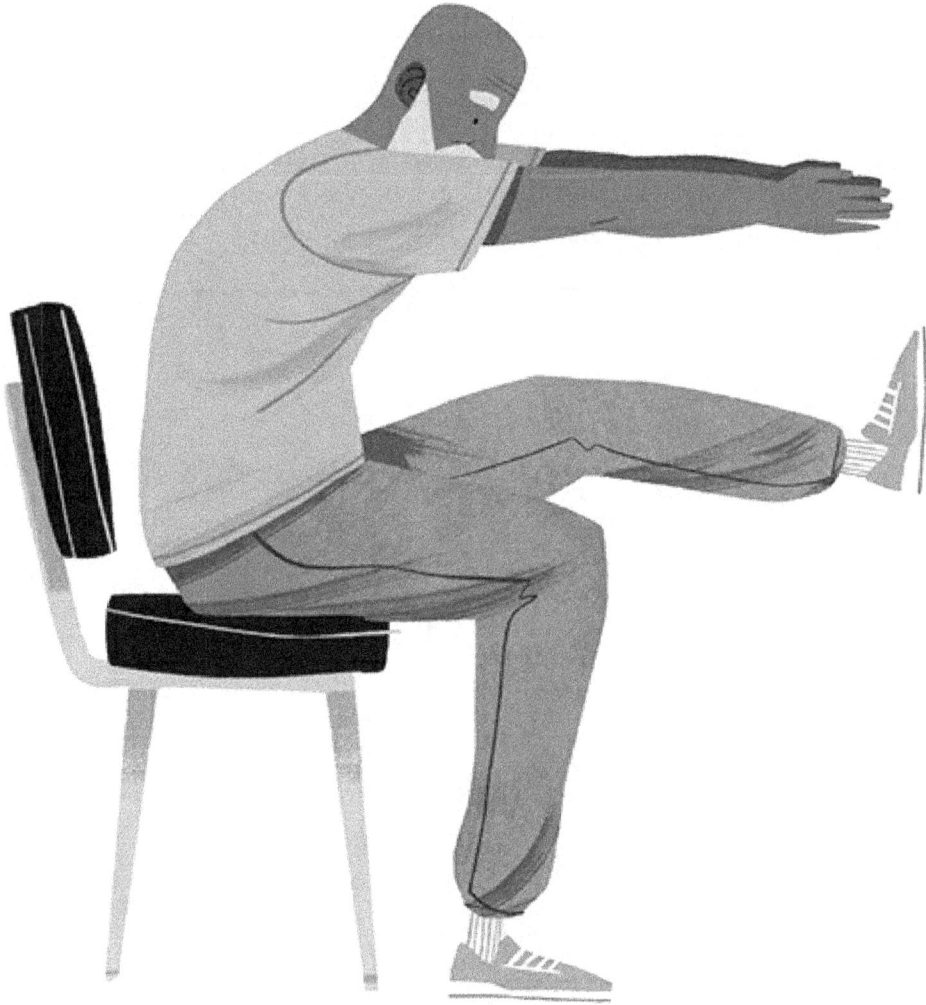

Straight Leg Crunch

Rectus abdominis   Transverse abdominis   Latissimus dorsi

In addition to working the core, this exercise builds strength in the hip flexors, which are essential for any activity that requires bending or kicking; even just walking uses these important muscles. If the hip flexors are weak, sudden movements can cause them to tear, which is a very painful injury.

INSTRUCTIONS

1   Begin in a seated position with your right leg extended straight out in front of you and your arms outstretched to either side. Inhale.

2   As you exhale, crunch forward, lifting your leg off the floor and bringing your arms to meet in front of you, reaching toward your foot.

3   Inhale as you return to the starting position. This is 1 rep. Aim for 8 to 10 reps, then do the other side.

Modification: Keep both feet on the ground to decrease the intensity, or add ankle weights to make this exercise more challenging.

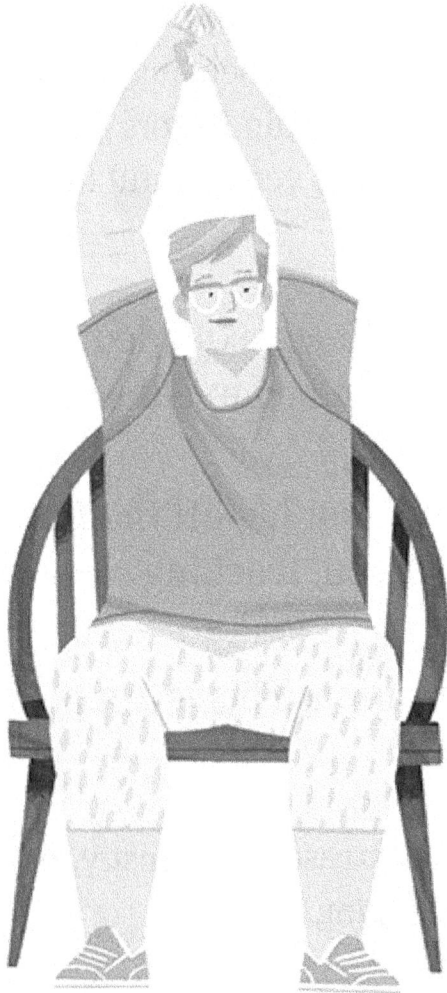

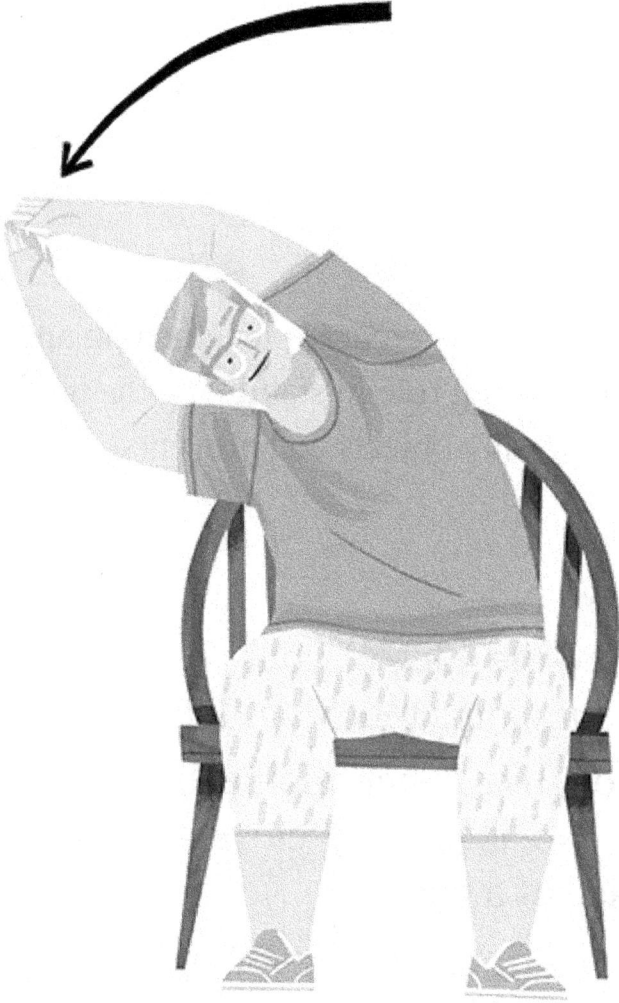

2

Metronome

Erector spinae / Obliques

The side-to-side movement of this exercise is great for lengthening and strengthening the obliques, which play a big role in stabilizing the trunk. A strong, stable trunk allows you to lift heavy objects and prevents hyperextension of the back.

INSTRUCTIONS

1. Begin sitting forward toward the edge of your chair, arms extended overhead with your palms touching. Inhale.

2. In a fluid, controlled motion, like a metronome, bend your torso to one side, then the other—to about 10 o'clock and 2 o'clock if you were looking at the face of a clock.

3. Breathe steadily as you move from side to side, maintaining the movement for 10 to 12 cycles of breath. Steady breath is more important than when you inhale and exhale.

Modification: To challenge your core strength, as you lean, lift your hip off the chair and hold for two seconds. Repeat on the other side.

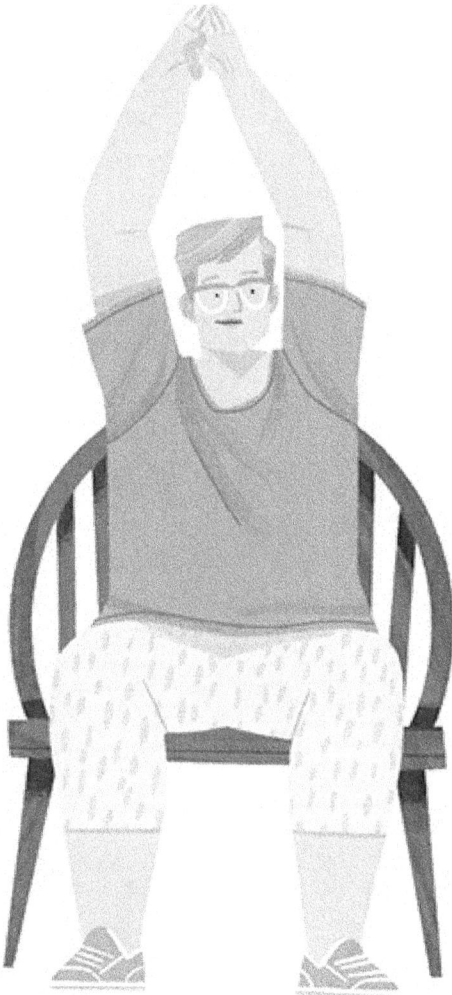

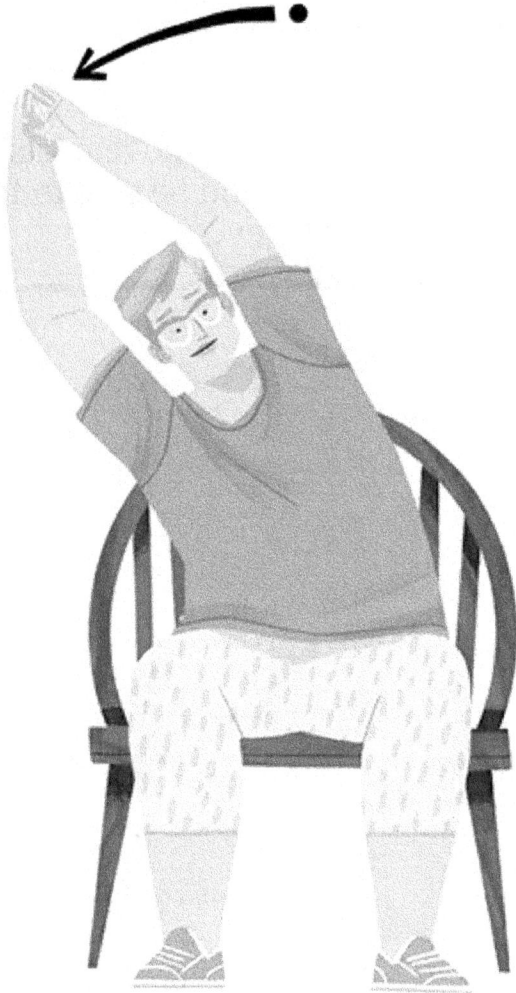

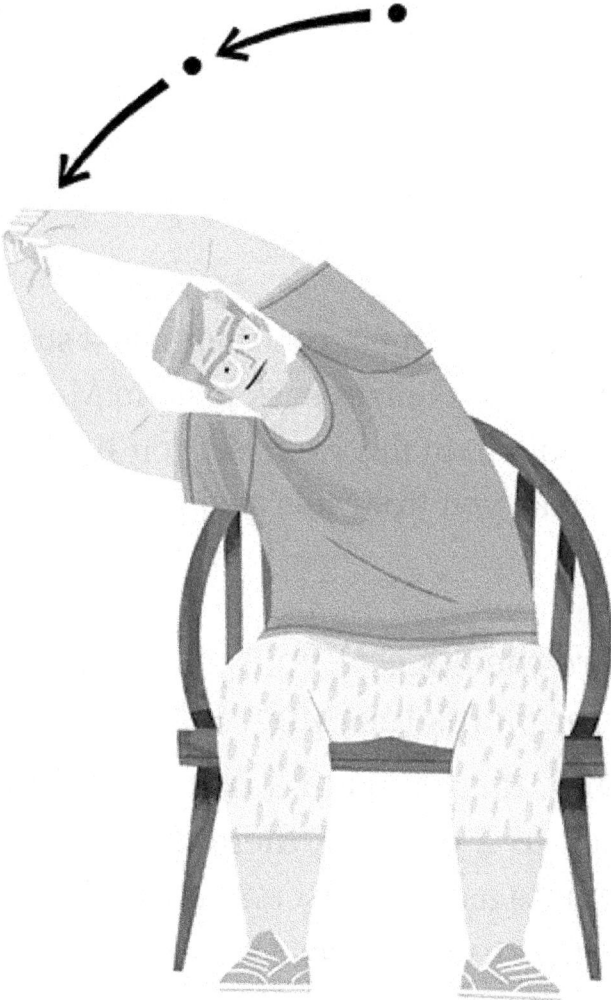

3

Ticking Clock

Erector spinae Obliques Rectus abdominis

Similar to the Metronome exercise, this movement contributes to a strong trunk, which also supports the spine and minimizes back pain. In Metronome, you move back and forth in a fluid motion. In this exercise, you'll use a series of tighter, controlled movements to take you from side to side.

INSTRUCTIONS

1   Begin sitting forward toward the edge of your chair, arms extended overhead with your palms touching. Inhale.

2   With your upper body, mimic the hands of a clock, "ticking" from 12 o'clock to 1 o'clock to 2 o'clock, then back to 1 o'clock and 12 o'clock. Exhale as you descend and inhale as you return to the top. Continue to the other side. This is 1 full rep.

3   Aim for 10 to 12 reps.

Modification: To increase the difficulty, add an additional stop at 3 o'clock on the right side and at 9 o'clock on the left.

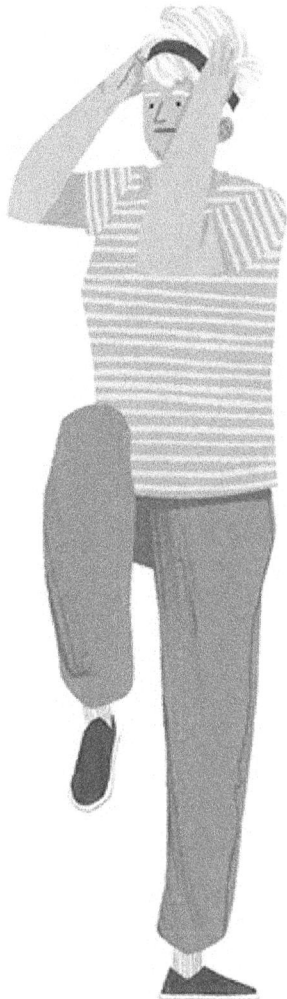

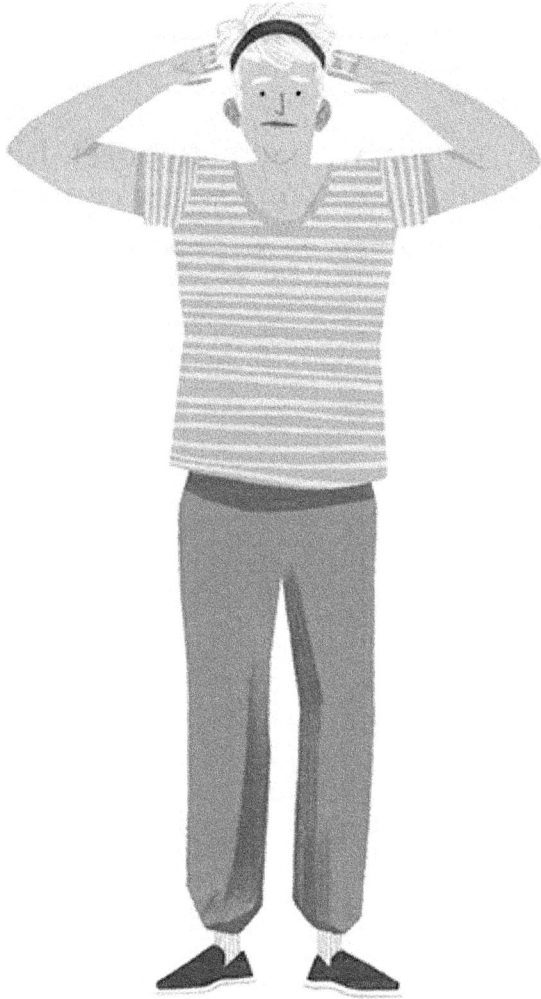

2

3

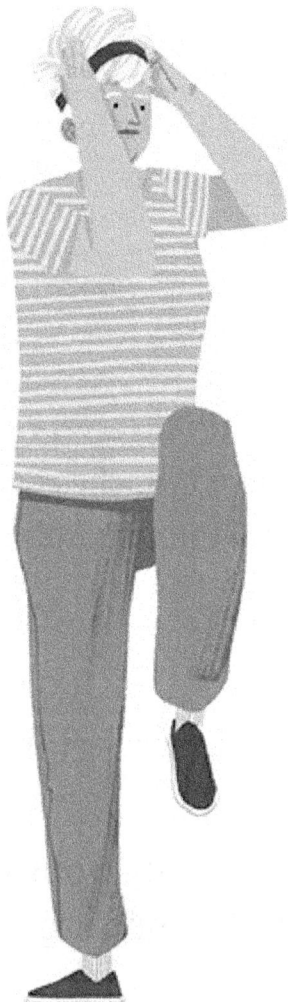

Standing Crunch

Transverse abdominis   Rectus abdominis   Obliques

Traditional crunches get a lot of hype, but they actually don't do a very good job of working the muscles deep within your core. Standing crunches do, helping build stability throughout your entire midsection while minimizing your risk of injury.

INSTRUCTIONS

1   Begin standing with your feet hip-width apart, hands behind your head. Inhale.

2   As you exhale, raise your right knee while crunching your left elbow across your body toward your knee. Pull your core inward.

3   Inhale as you return to the starting position. Repeat on the other side. This is 1 rep.

4   Aim to complete a set of 20 reps.

Modification: For less intensity, perform the crunch without lifting your knee. For more intensity, add reps or try adding ankle weights.

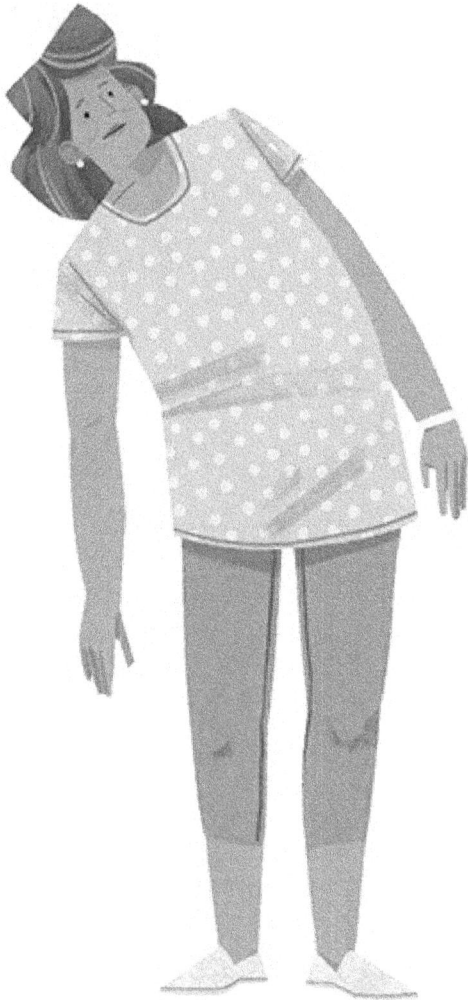

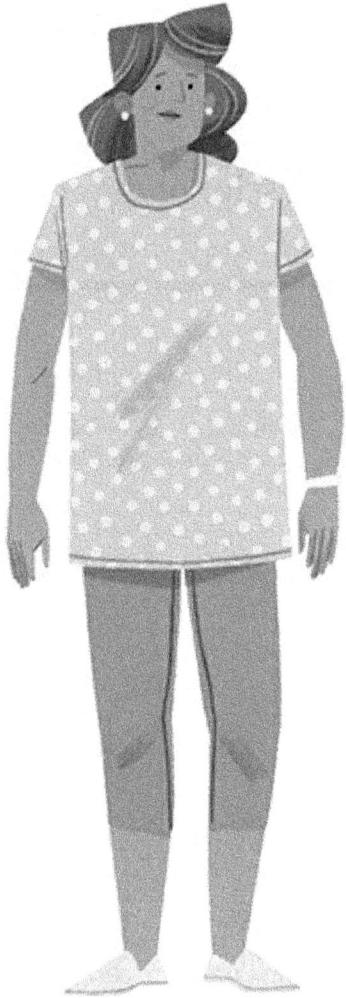

2

3

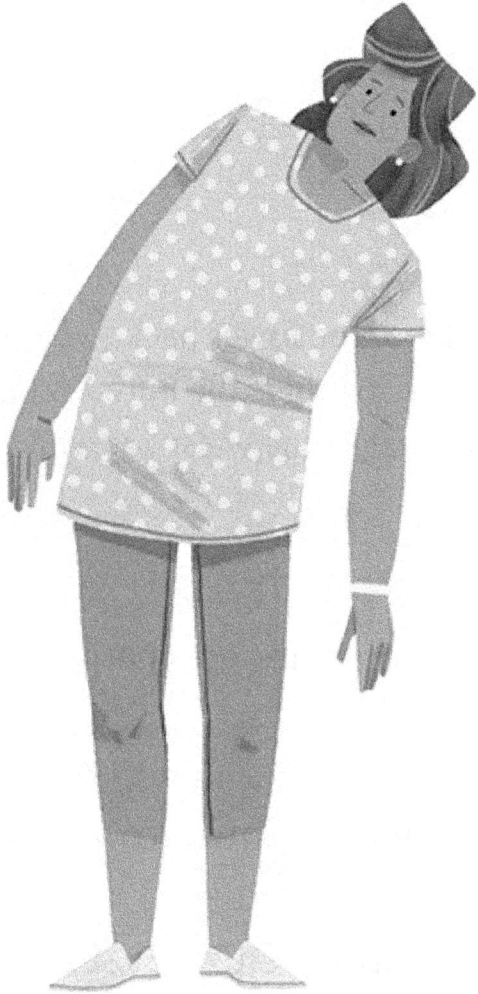

Side Bends

Obliques   Erector spinae

This move increases the strength and flexibility of the lower back, which will help keep you from throwing your back out. It also builds the muscles that support the spine, promotes good posture and sculpts the waist . . . who doesn't love that?

INSTRUCTIONS

1   Begin standing with your feet hip-width apart, arms at your sides, and a gentle bend in your knees. Inhale.

2   As you exhale, contract your side abdominal wall and bend to the right side, reaching your right fingertips down toward the floor.

3   Inhale as you return to the starting position. This is 1 rep. Aim for 10 to 15 reps on both sides.

Modification: To increase the difficulty, hold a dumbbell in each hand. You can also perform this exercise while clasping your hands overhead in a motion similar to that of the Metronome exercise.

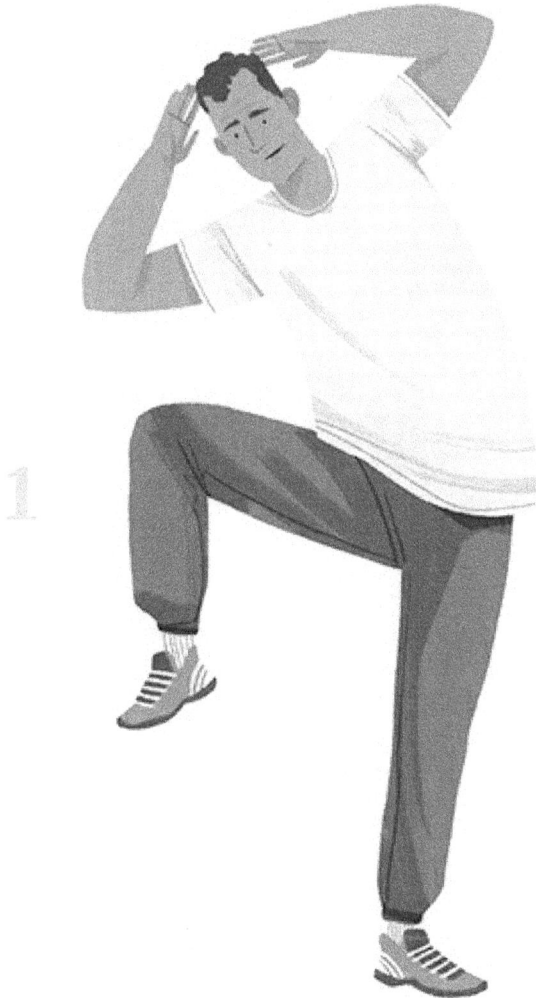

1

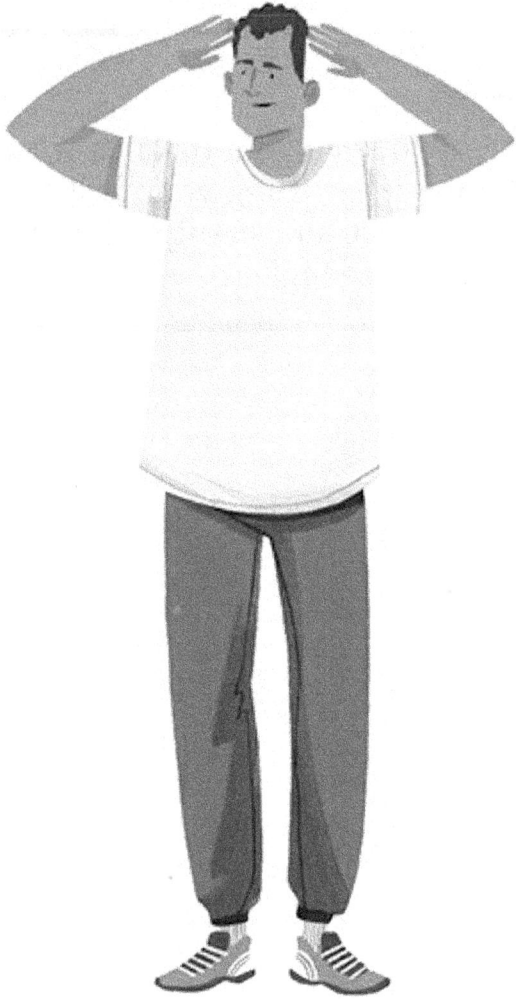

2

3

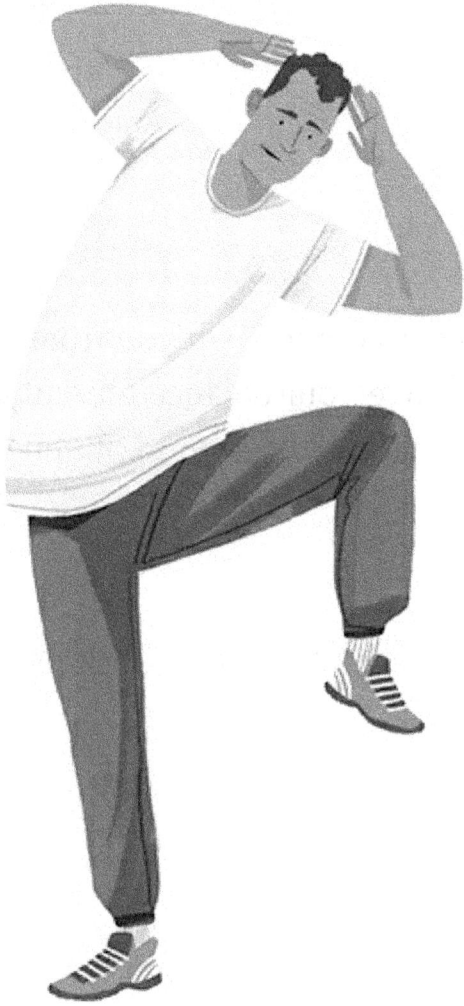

Side Crunch with Leg Lift

Obliques / Erector spinae

Anytime you bend at the waist, you rely on your core to keep you from toppling over. These exercises will really improve your balance for daily life, so you can easily retrieve that item you dropped, or bend over to put on your shoes without having to sit down.

INSTRUCTIONS

1   Begin by standing with your feet hip-width apart, hands behind your head. Inhale.

2   As you exhale, open your right hip and raise your right knee to the side of your body. At the same time, crunch your right elbow down to meet your knee.

3   Inhale as you return to the starting position. This is 1 rep. Aim for 8 reps on each side.

Modification: For less intensity, perform the crunch while keeping both feet on the floor. For more intensity, add reps or try adding ankle weights.

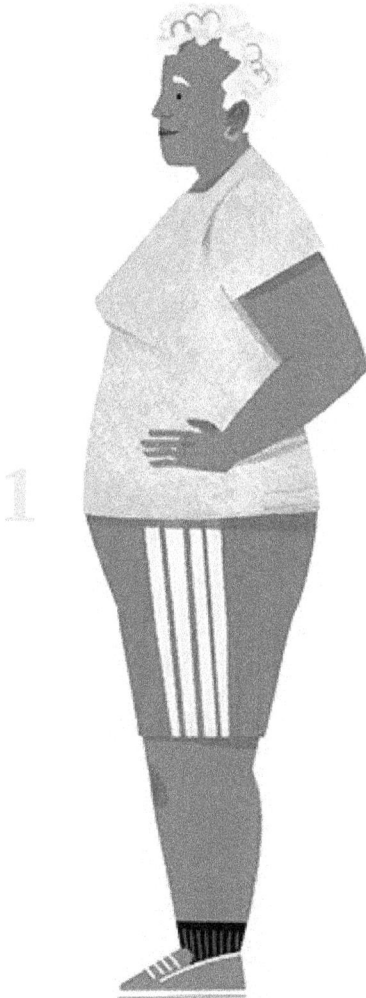

1

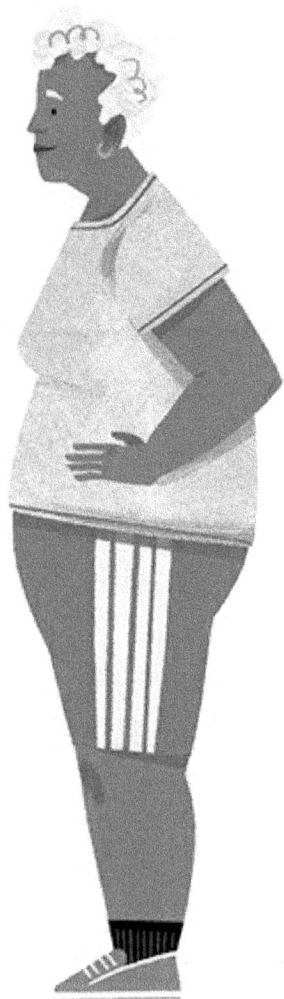

Pelvic Tilt

Rectus abdominis   Transverse abdominis   Obliques

This exercise engages your core and hip muscles in tandem. These are the same muscle groups you use to stand comfortably without pain and to bend over and touch your toes. Any type of deadlift move—that is, bending over and picking up an object off the floor in front of you—requires these muscles to be strong and functioning properly.

INSTRUCTIONS

1   Stand up straight and tall with your hands on your hips, feet about shoulder-width apart, and a gentle bend in your knees. Inhale.

2   As you exhale, contract your abdominal muscles and tilt your pelvis forward, making a concave shape with your chest. Your shoulders may come forward slightly as well.

3   Inhale as you return to the neutral position. This is 1 rep. Aim for 15 to 20 reps.

Modification: When you are first getting started, you may find it helpful to do this exercise with your back against a wall, so you can feel the difference between the "neutral" and "engaged" positions.

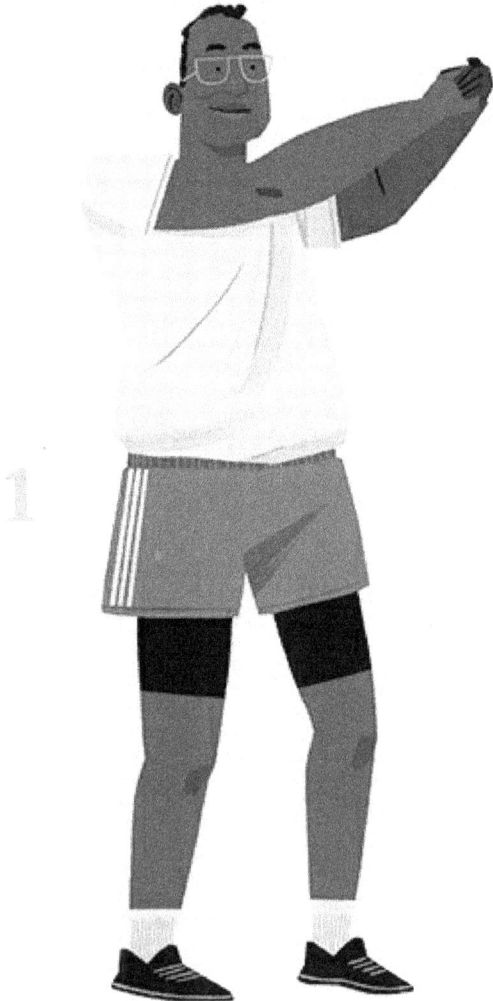

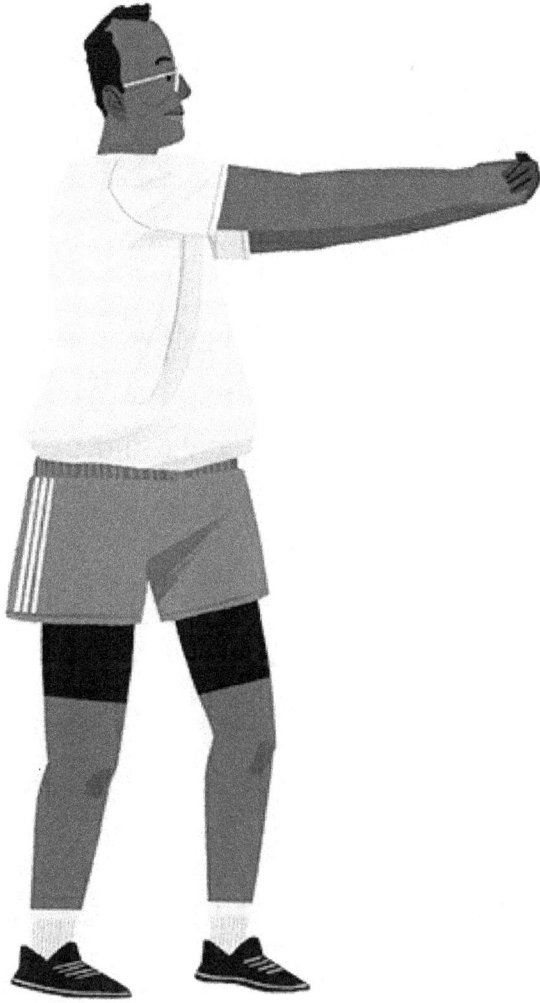

2

Torso Twists

Rectus abdominis   Transverse abdominis   Obliques   Erector spinae

Working on your golf swing? You'll love this exercise. Even if you're not a golfer, being able to comfortably rotate your torso is key to so many movements you do in daily life. These twists build the muscles that protect the spine, preventing back injuries.

INSTRUCTIONS

1   Begin with your feet hip-width apart, arms extended in front of you at shoulder level with your hands clasped. Inhale.

2   Engage your core and exhale as you twist to one side, looking in the direction you're twisting.

3   Return to center as you inhale and twist to the opposite side as you exhale. This is 1 rep. Aim for 10 to 15 reps.

Modification: For more of a challenge, hold a kettlebell, medicine ball, or dumbbell while you perform the move.

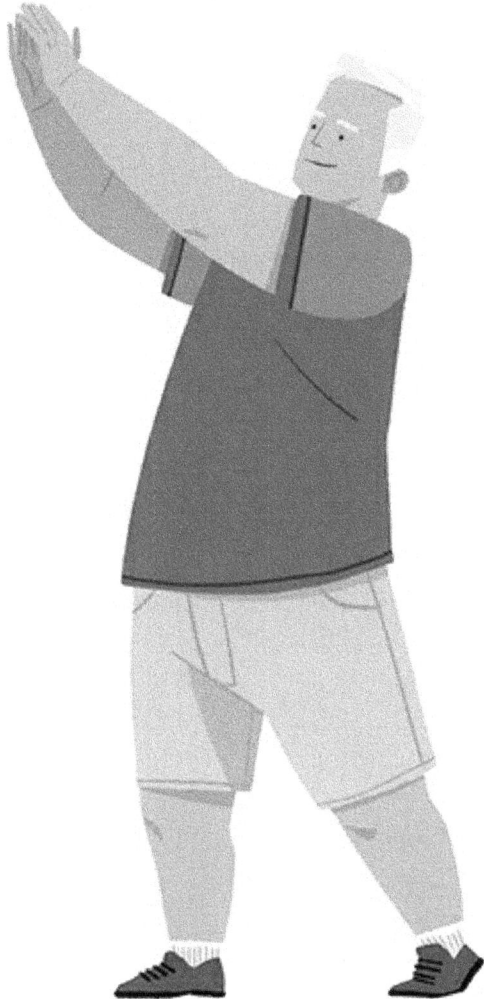

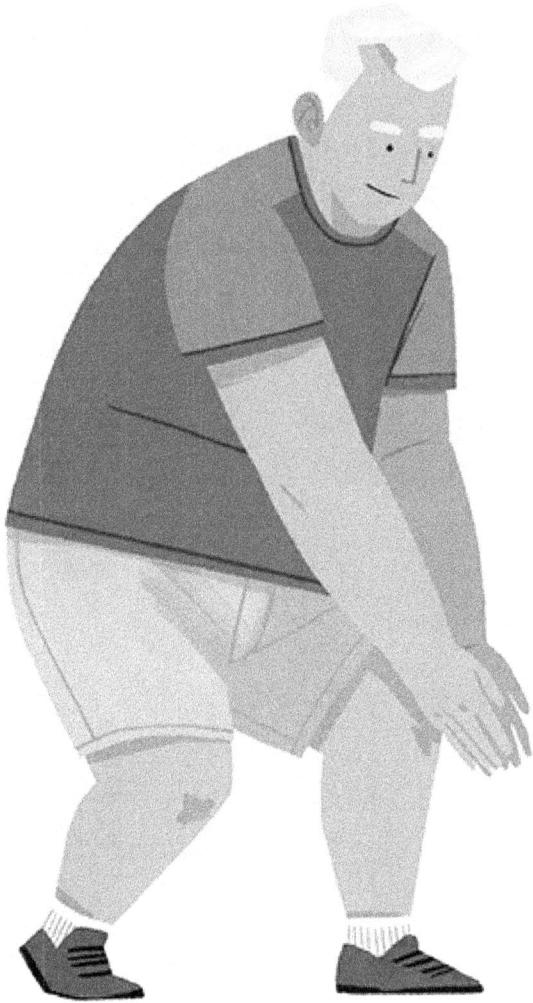

Wood Chop

Transverse abdominis Obliques Latissimus dorsi

If you play any sport involving a racket, such as tennis, racquetball, or pickleball, this exercise will improve your game. It promotes a strong range of motion and improves the flexibility of the spine.

INSTRUCTIONS

1 Stand with your feet slightly wider than hip-width apart, hands clasped in front of you with your arms straight.

2 As you inhale, reach your arms up diagonally to the right side, pivoting your hips toward the right and positioning the majority of your weight on your right foot.

3 As you exhale, bring your arms downward and diagonally across your body in a chopping motion. Bend at the waist and twist down toward your left, shifting your weight to your left foot. End with your hands just outside your left shin.

4 This is 1 rep. Aim for 10 to 12 reps on the right, then do the left side.

Modification: For more of a challenge, hold a kettlebell, medicine ball, or dumbbell while you perform the move.

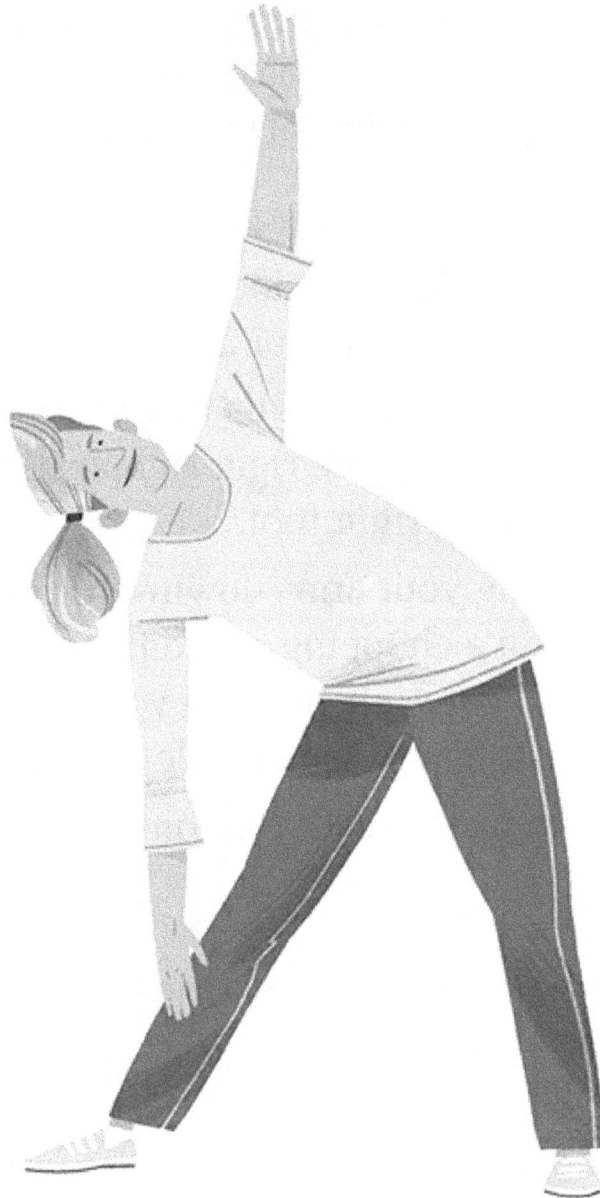

Triangle

Rectus abdominis   Transverse abdominis   Obliques   Latissimus dorsi

If you practice yoga, you may know this pose by its Sanskrit name, *trikonasana*. It's an all-around great core strengthener, improving the flexibility of the spine, relieving tension in the back, opening the hips, and stretching the hamstrings.

INSTRUCTIONS

1   Begin in a standing position with your feet wider than hip-width apart.

2   Turn your right toes outward so that they point to the right. As you inhale, raise your arms until they extend out to your sides at shoulder level.

3   Pulling your belly button toward your spine, engage your core, and bend sideways at the waist as you exhale, lowering your right hand down toward your outer right shin.

4   Hold this pose for three to four cycles of breath. Then activate your core and return to a standing position. Repeat on the other side. One pose on each side is enough.

Modification: To make the pose easier, bring your hand to your thigh rather than your shin. For more of a challenge, try bringing your hand all the way to the floor.

REMEMBER

When doing this move correctly, you'll also feel your glutes working as you sit back into your rear hip.

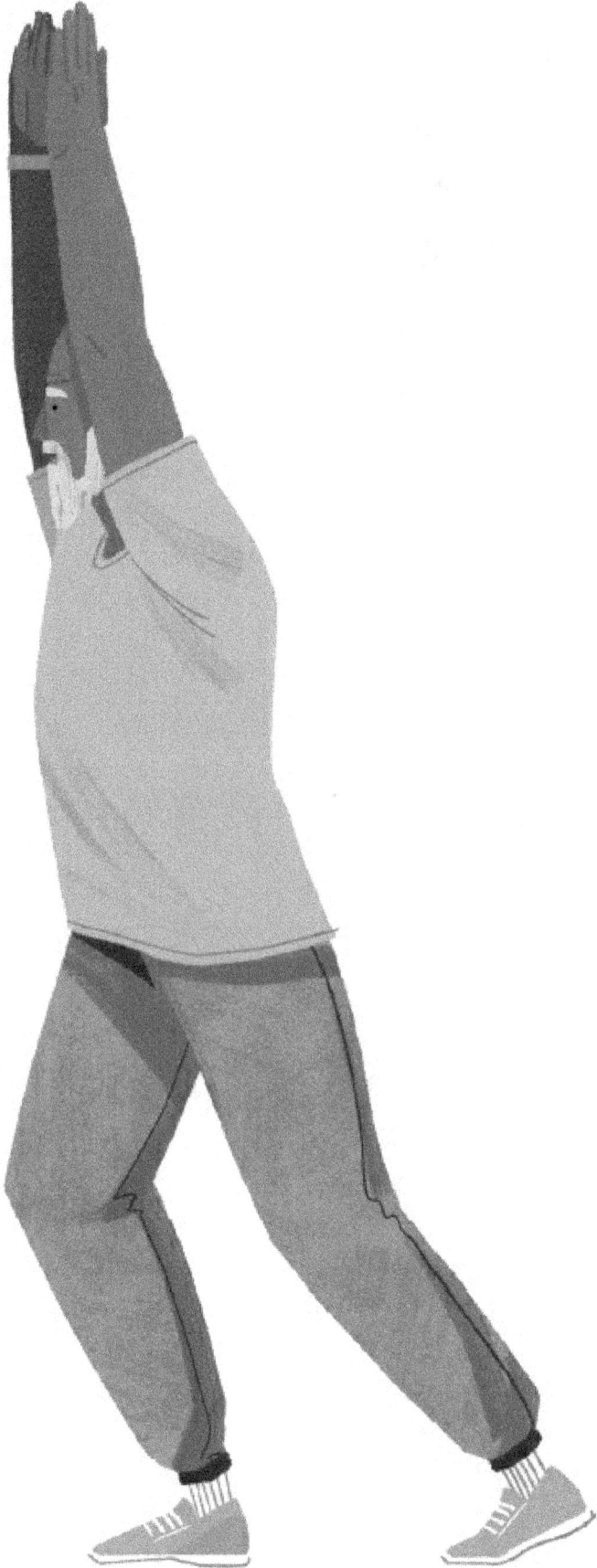

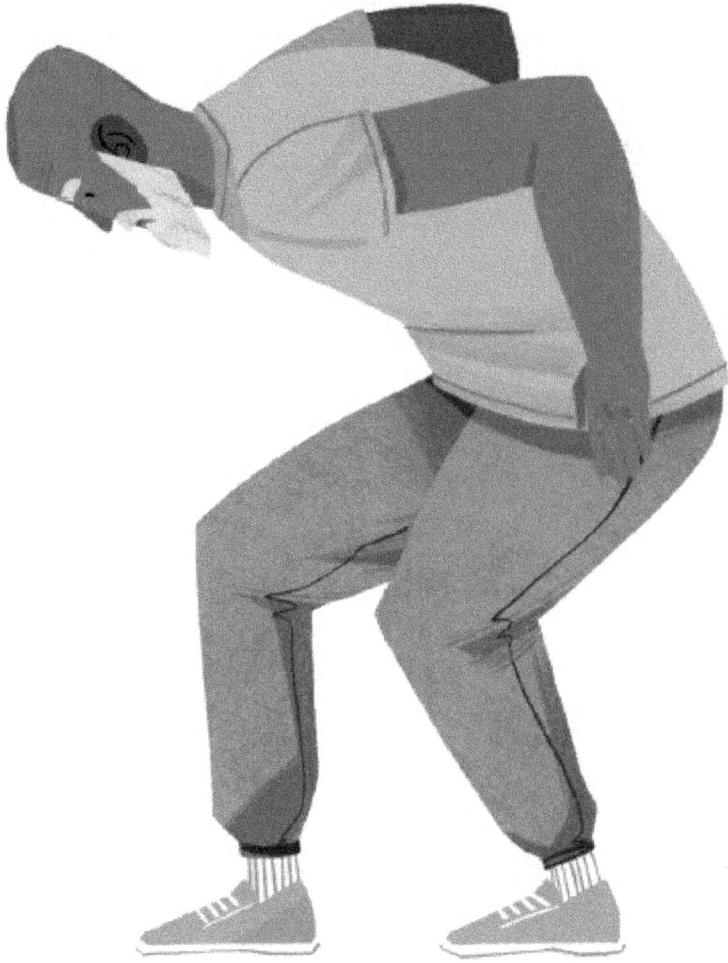

Diagonal Sit Back

This exercise mimics the motion of reaching up for an object on a high shelf, which is definitely not a time when you want to falter. This two-in-one move will improve your balance while also strengthening your core.

INSTRUCTIONS

1. Begin in a standing position. Angle your body slightly toward the right, the toes of your left and right feet pointing in the same direction as your shoulders.

2. Inhale while reaching both arms up toward the right corner, shifting your weight to your front foot.

3. As you exhale, engage your core and bend forward at the waist, bringing your arms to your sides and sitting back into your left hip. Your weight should shift onto your back foot, with your back knee slightly bent.

4. Return to the upright position. This is 1 rep. Aim for 10 to 12 reps, then repeat on the other side.

Modification: To test your core strength and balance, as you lift forward to the corner, raise your back foot off the ground behind you and reach higher, elongating the core even more before continuing back into the crunch position.

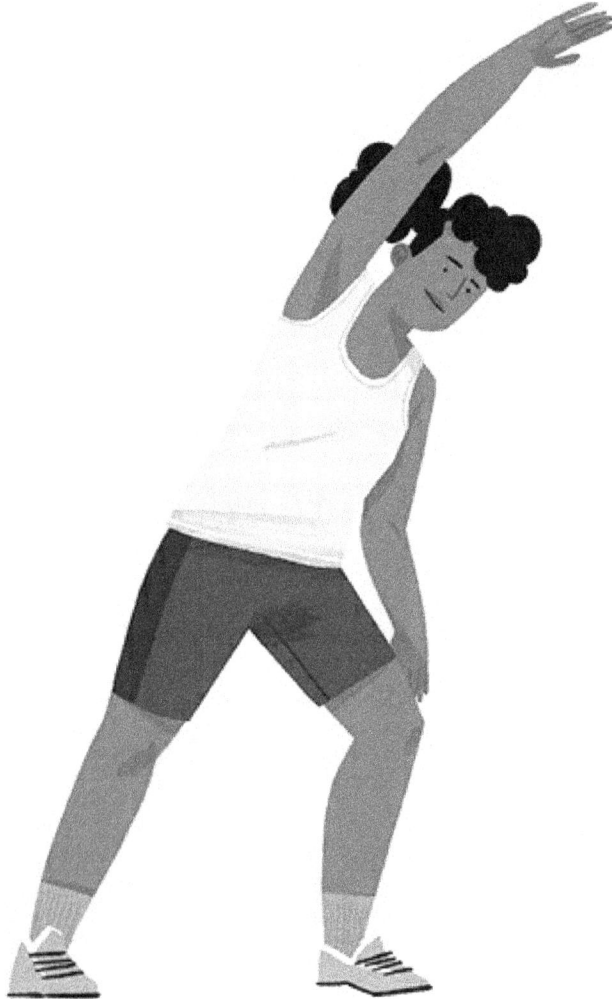

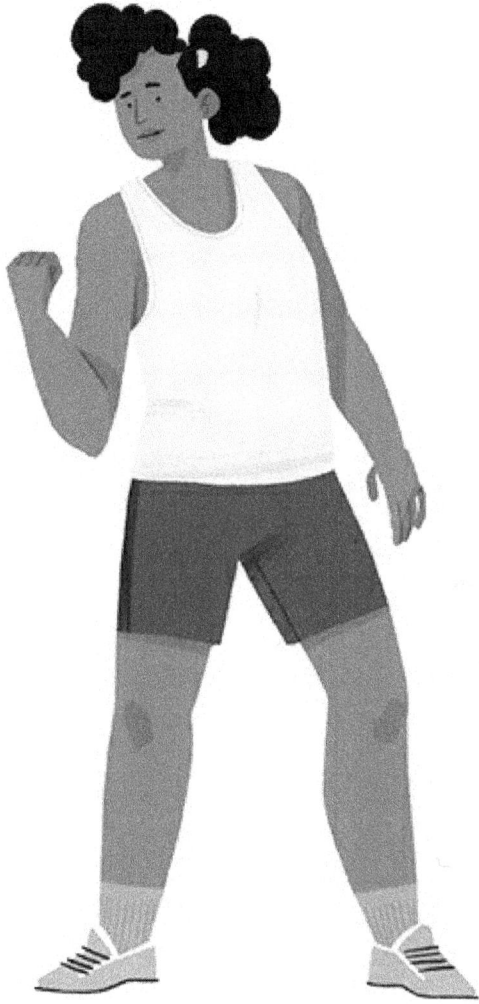

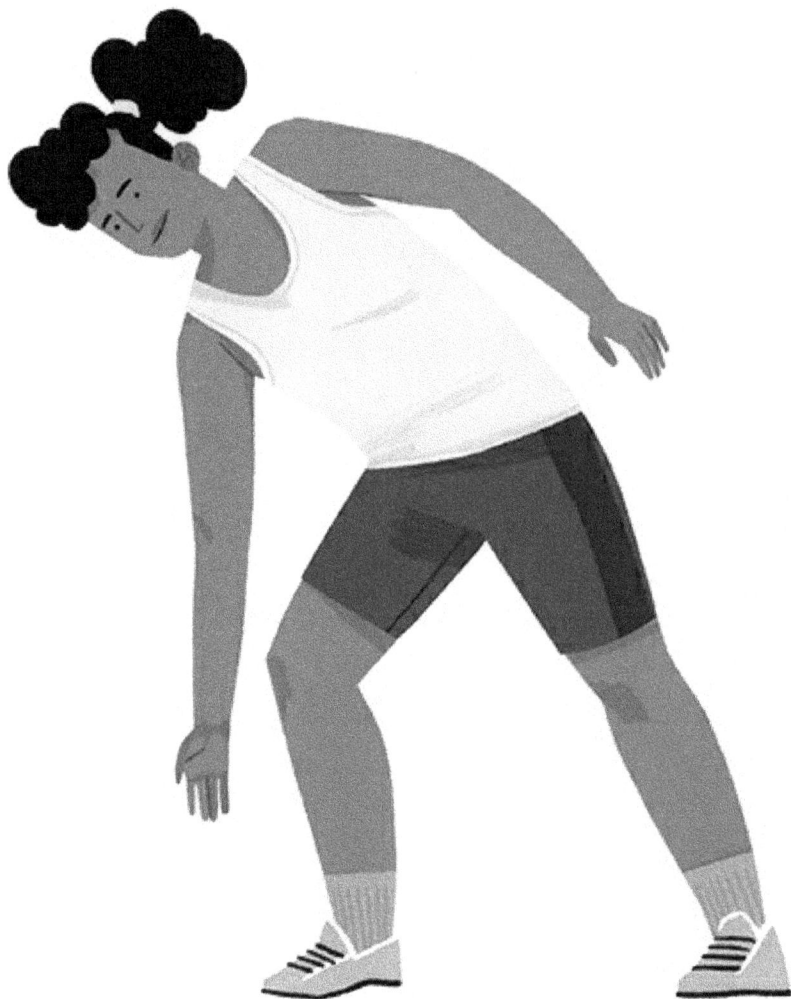

Lunging Pull-Down

Rectus abdominis / Transverse abdominis / Latissimus dorsi / Obliques

This is a great move for building the muscles you use anytime you work on something overhead, such as pulling the cord on a ceiling fan, reaching up to change a lightbulb, or closing a sash window. It also targets those pesky love handles!

INSTRUCTIONS

1 Begin in a standing position with your feet wider than hip-width apart. Turn your toes outward slightly. Keep your feet in the same position throughout.

2 Inhale as you lunge to the right, reaching your left arm up overhead in the direction of your lunge and right by your ear.

3 As you exhale, tighten your core and move back through center to a lunge on the left side, bending at the waist and bringing your left elbow down toward your hip, and continue down reaching your left hand down to your left ankle.

4 This is 1 rep. Aim for 10 to 12 reps, then perform the exercise on the other side.

Modification: To reduce the difficulty, bring your arm to your knee or thigh rather than your ankle on the downward motion.

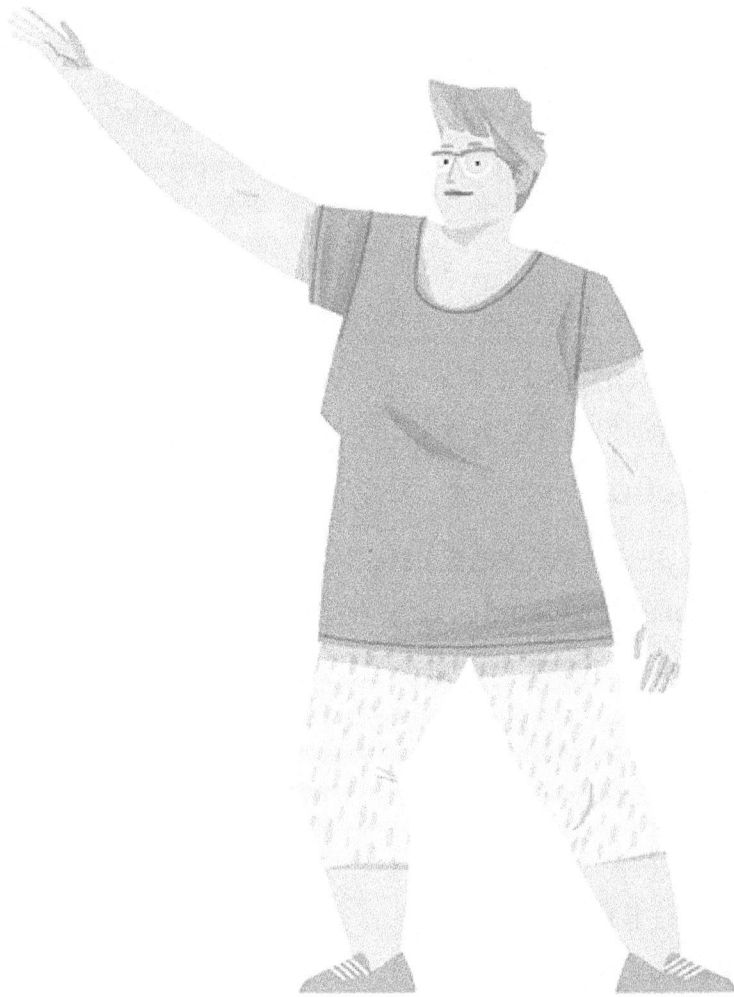

1

2

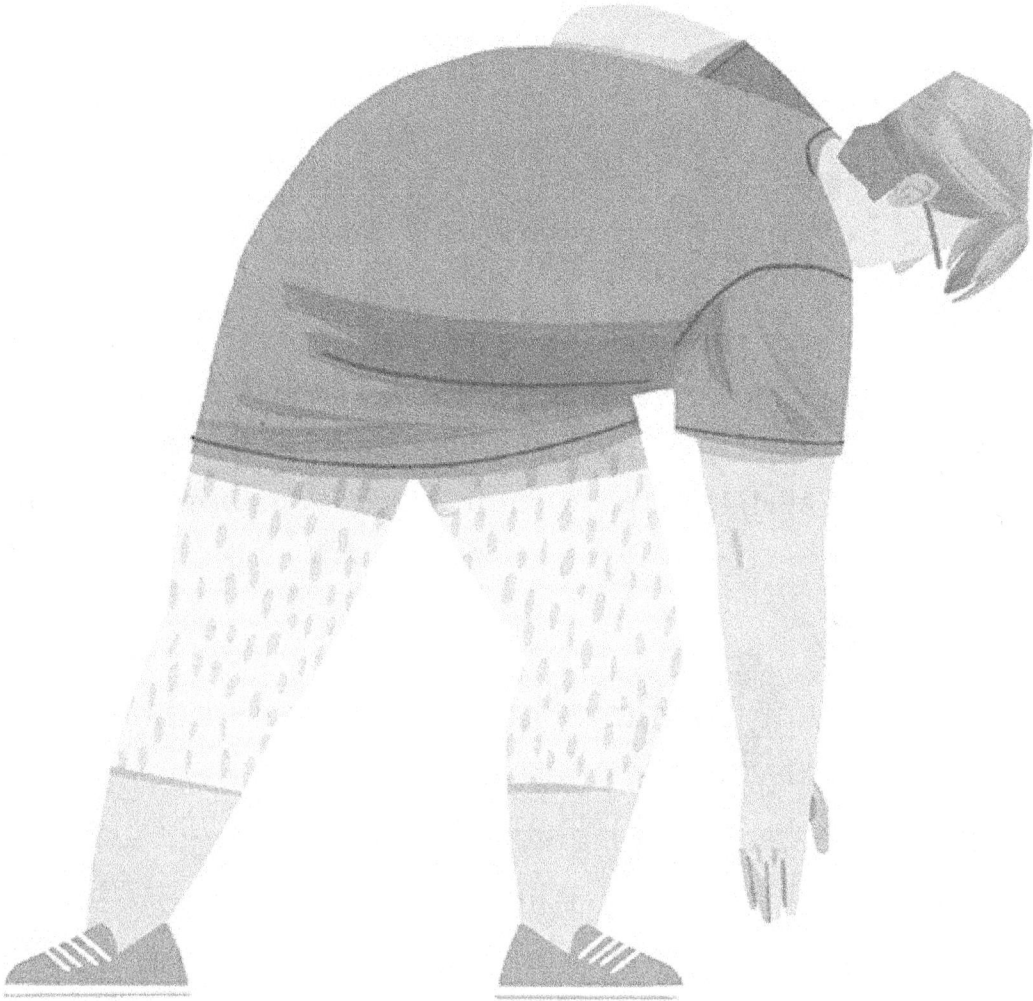

Cross Pull-Down

Rectus abdominis / Transverse abdominis / Latissimus dorsi

In addition to working the core, this move will help you maintain a wide range of motion in the shoulders and arms, which, believe it or not, play an important role in stopping falls. Think of what happens when you start to lose your balance; without even thinking about it, you stick an arm out to steady yourself.

INSTRUCTIONS

1   Begin in a standing position with your feet wider than hip-width apart. Turn your toes outward slightly.

2   Inhale as you lunge to the right, reaching your right arm up overhead in the direction of your lunge.

3   As you exhale, engage your core and move back through center to a lunge on the left side, bending at the waist and bringing your right arm down and across your body toward your left ankle.

4   This is 1 rep. Aim for 10 to 12 reps, then perform the exercise on the other side.

Modification: To reduce the difficulty, bring your arm to your knee or thigh rather than your ankle on the downward motion.

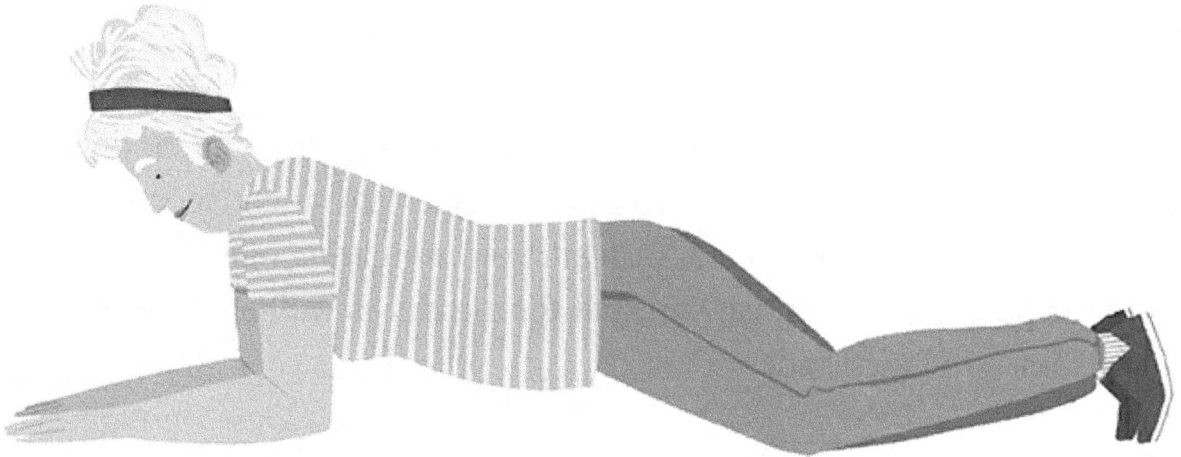

Kneeling Plank

Rectus abdominis / Transverse abdominis

This exercise proves that you don't have to lift heavy weights or do high-impact moves to get a firm core. This is an isometric exercise, meaning there's no movement involved. Instead, you're fighting against gravity to hold the position. It's a great workout for the abs as well as the arms, shoulders, and lower back.

INSTRUCTIONS

1   Begin on all fours with your hands directly underneath your shoulders. Place your elbows where your palms are, so your forearms are flat on the mat.

2   Slowly walk your knees out behind you to bring your torso into a straight line, your belly suspended over the mat.

3   Keeping the spine straight, tighten your abdominal muscles and hold the pose, breathing in and out. Work up to holding the pose for 30 seconds.

Modification: If you can hold your kneeling plank with proper form for 30 seconds and are looking for more of a challenge, move on to a traditional plank with your knees raised off the ground.

1

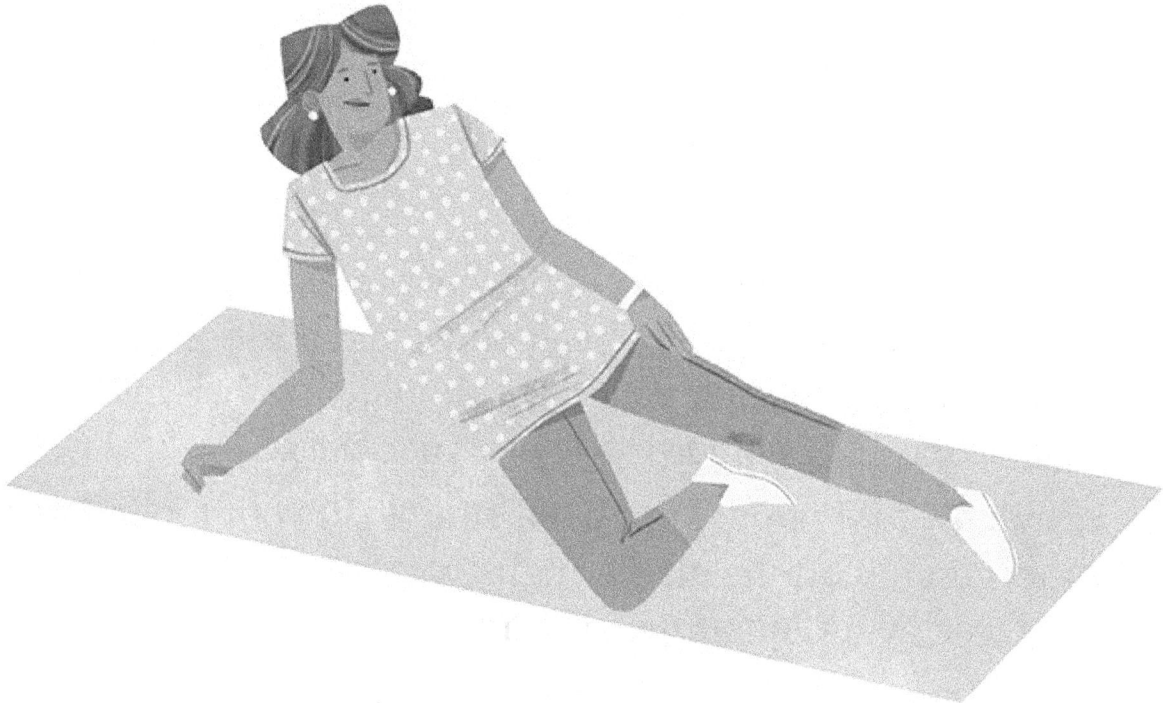

2

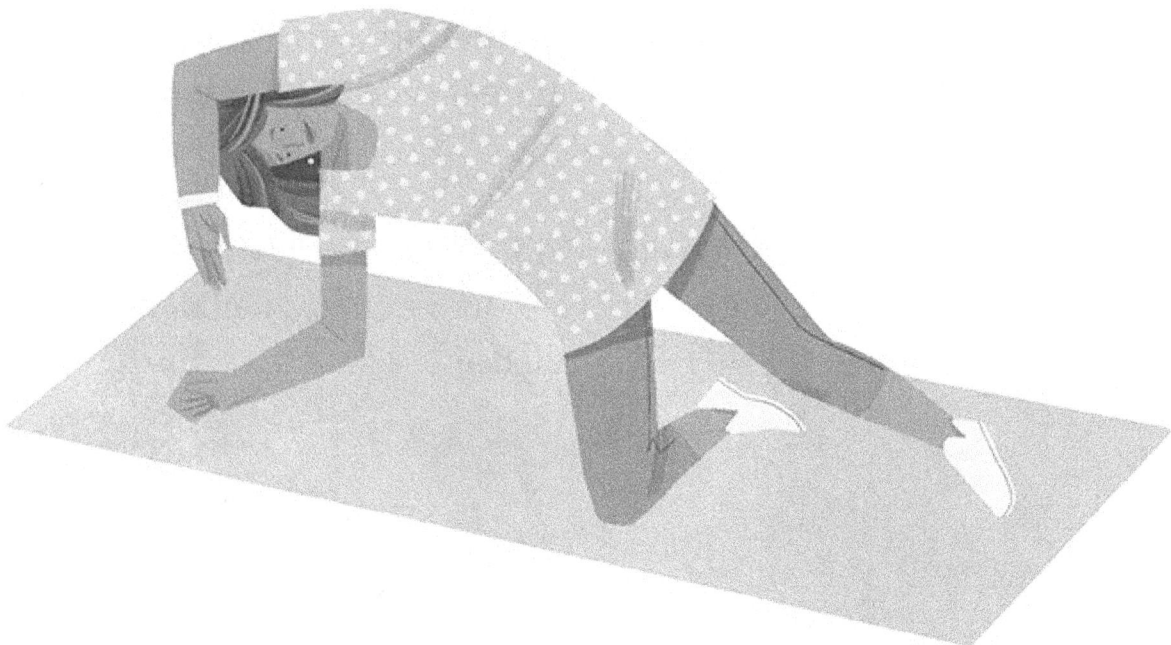

Modified Side Plank

TARGET MUSCLE GROUP

Obliques

Like the Kneeling Plank, this exercise does a lot of work without you doing a whole lot of movement. This exercise, combined with the Kneeling Plank, will help pull your midsection in like a corset, defining your waist and strengthening your whole core.

INSTRUCTIONS

1. Begin by sitting on the mat with your weight on your right hip, legs bent to your left side. Lean down and position your right elbow directly beneath your right shoulder so that your forearm rests on the mat, supporting your upper body.

2. Keeping your bottom knee bent, straighten your top leg and lift your right hip off the mat, bringing your torso in line with your hip. Reach your left arm overhead.

3. Engage your core and hold the pose, breathing in and out and being mindful not to drop your right hip. Work up to holding the pose for 30 seconds, then repeat on the other side. Once on each side is enough.

Modification: If you can hold your modified side plank with proper form for 30 seconds and want more of a challenge, move on to a traditional side plank with your bottom leg straight rather than bent.

1

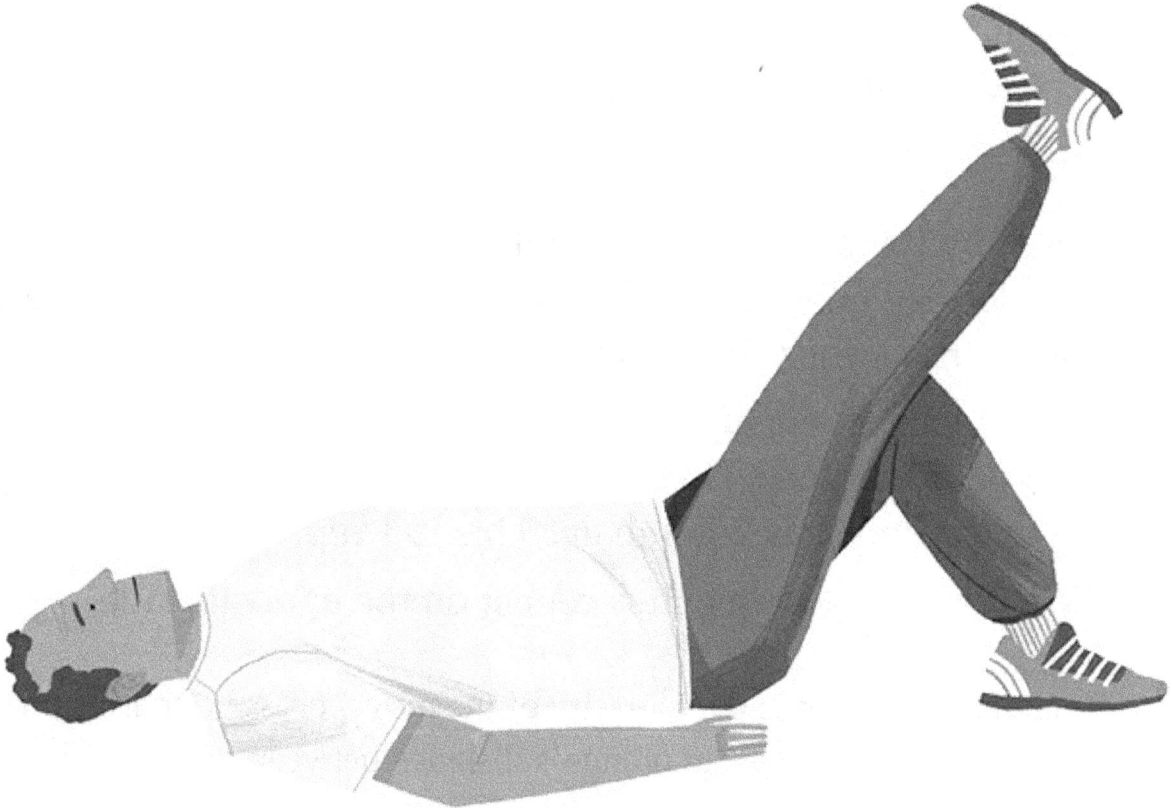

2

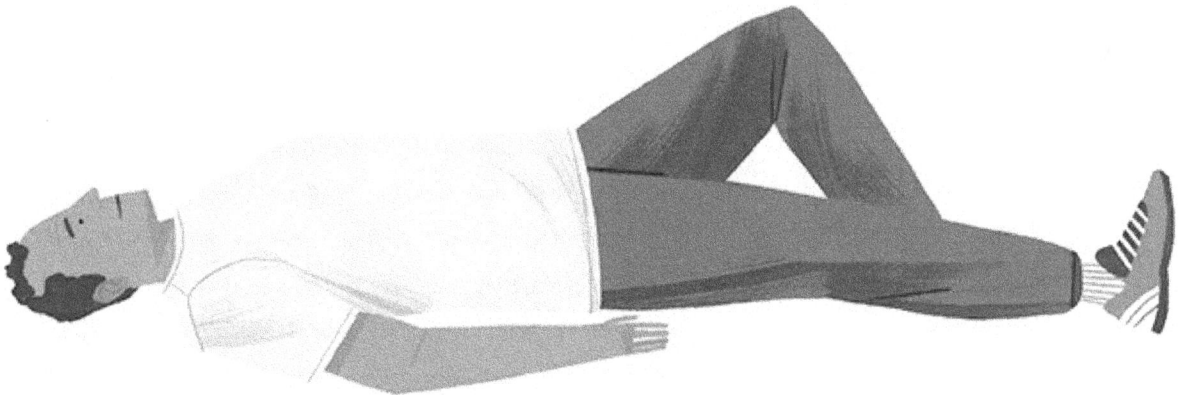

Single Leg Lifts

Rectus abdominis / Obliques

Although your leg is doing the moving in this exercise, you'll need to engage your core to stabilize the rest of your body, which translates to a stable core for everyday activities such as carrying groceries.

INSTRUCTIONS

1. Begin by lying on your back with your right leg straight and your left leg bent so your left foot is flat on the ground. Relax your arms at your sides. Inhale.

2. As you exhale, engage your core and lift your right leg in line with your left knee. Hold for 2 seconds, then lower your right leg with control as you inhale. This is 1 rep.

3. Aim for 10 to 12 reps, then repeat on the opposite side.

Modification: To increase the intensity of the move, cross your arms on your chest, remembering to keep an orange's distance between your chin and your chest.

REMEMBER

This doesn't need to be a huge crunching motion. Even a small crunch, when engaging your abs properly, will provide noticeable results. Proper form is most important.

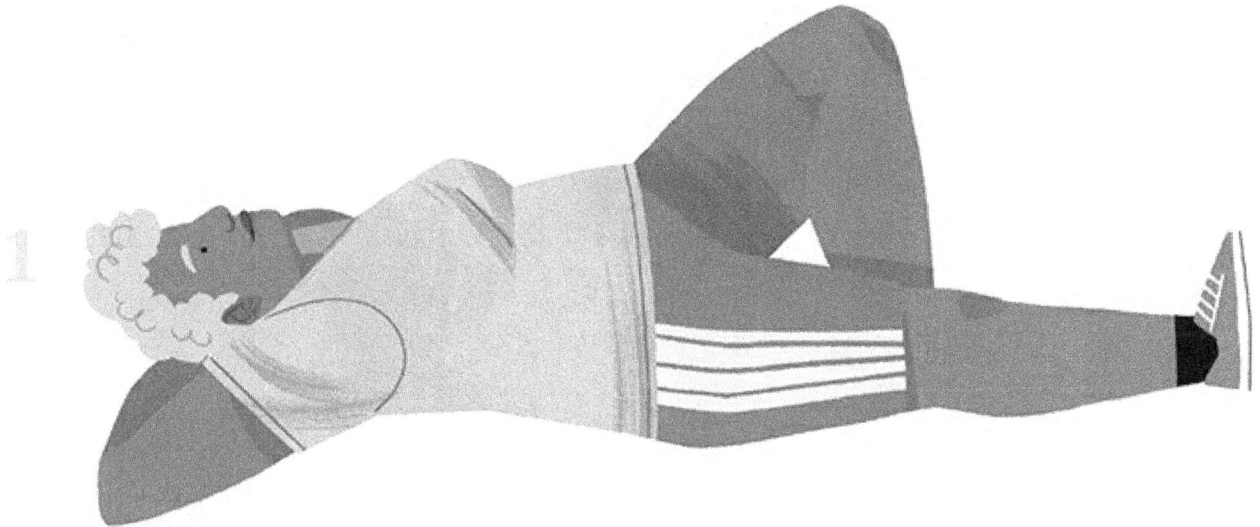

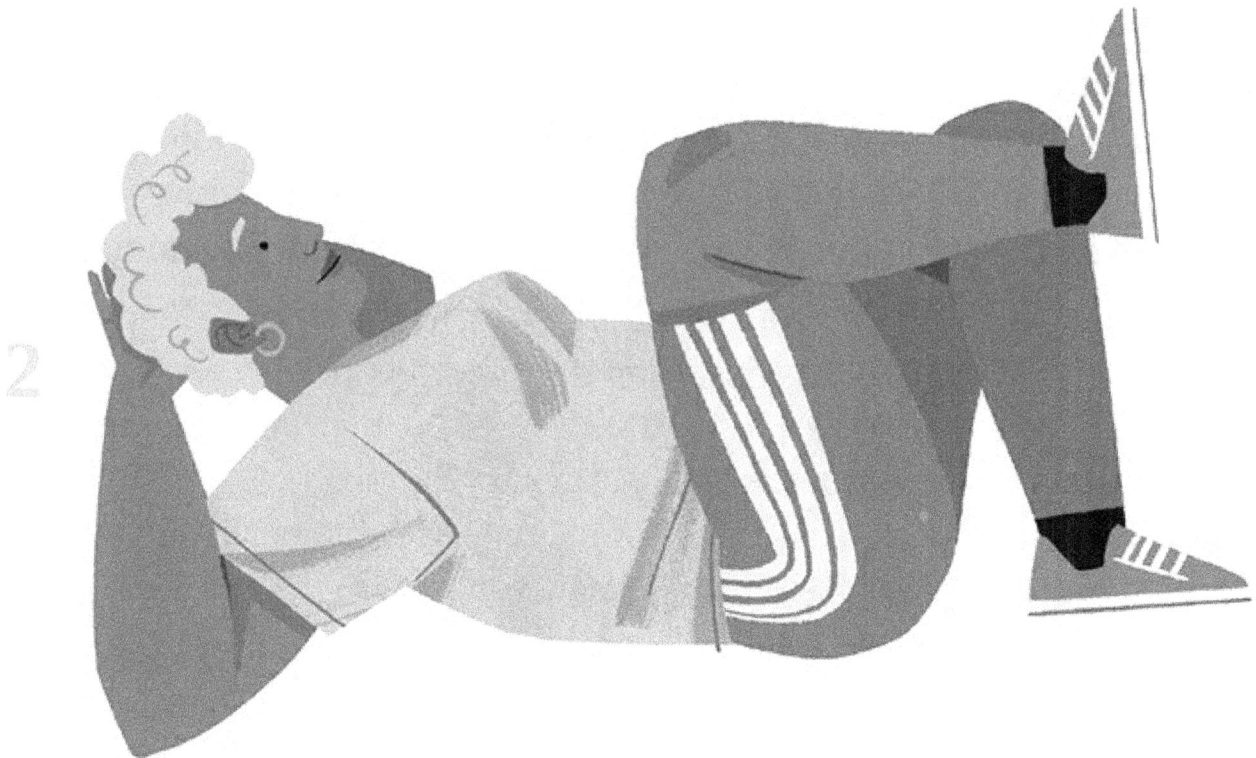

One-Legged Crunch

Rectus abdominis Transverse abdominis

Aside from the increased likelihood of injury from performing them, traditional crunches are not the preferred option because it's too easy to breeze through them without engaging the core muscles in an effective way. By incorporating a leg into the move, you're forcing the whole core to engage, working the midsection in a way that dozens of regular crunches can't.

INSTRUCTIONS

1   Begin by lying on your back with your right leg straight and your left leg bent so your left foot is flat on the ground. Place your hands behind your head. Inhale.

2   As you exhale, bend your right knee and raise your head off the mat, crunching toward the center. Don't tuck your chin to your chest. Instead, imagine holding an orange between your chin and your chest—this is how much space you should maintain.

3   Inhale as you lower your right leg back to the floor. This is 1 rep. Aim for 10 to 12 reps, then do the other side.

Modification: To increase the difficulty, stretch your arms overhead by your ears and maintain as you crunch up. Avoid bringing the arms forward, which uses momentum. Instead, keep your arms by your ears so they act like a stabilizer and add resistance.

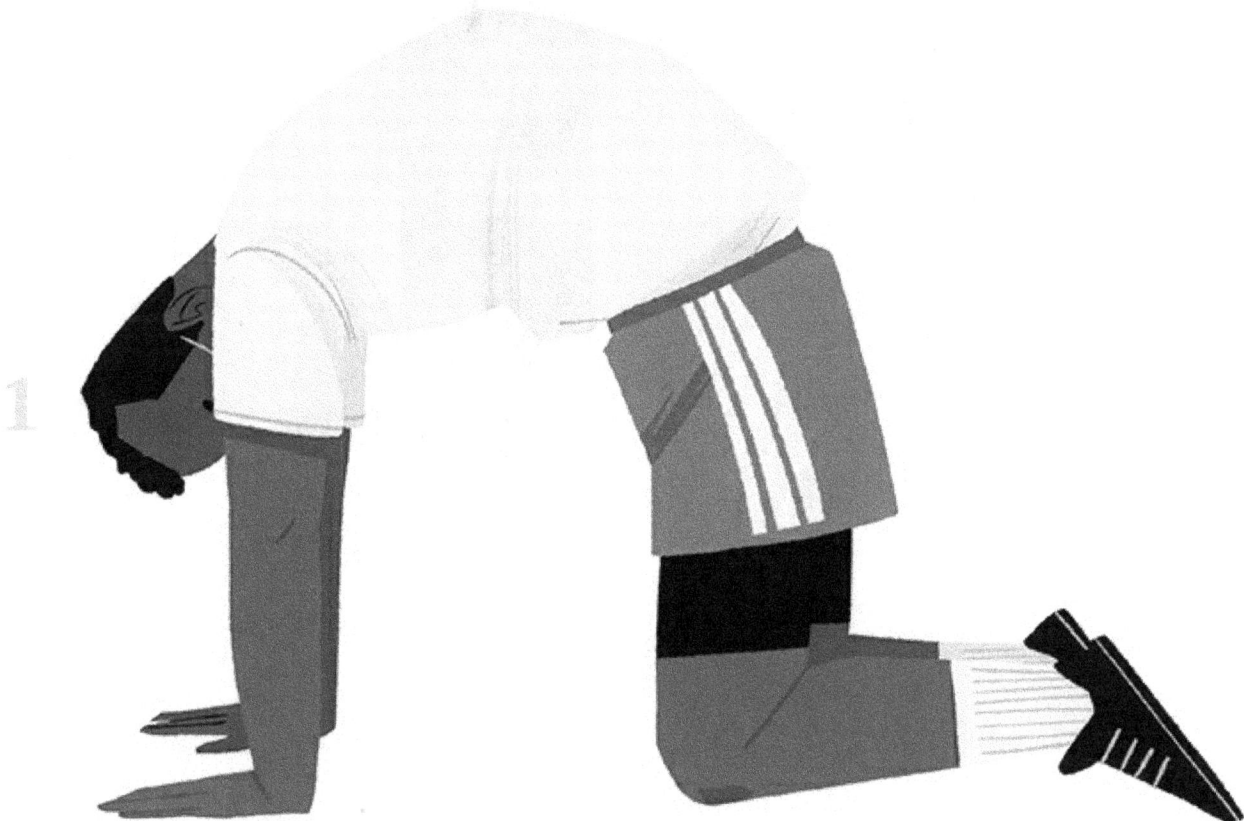

1

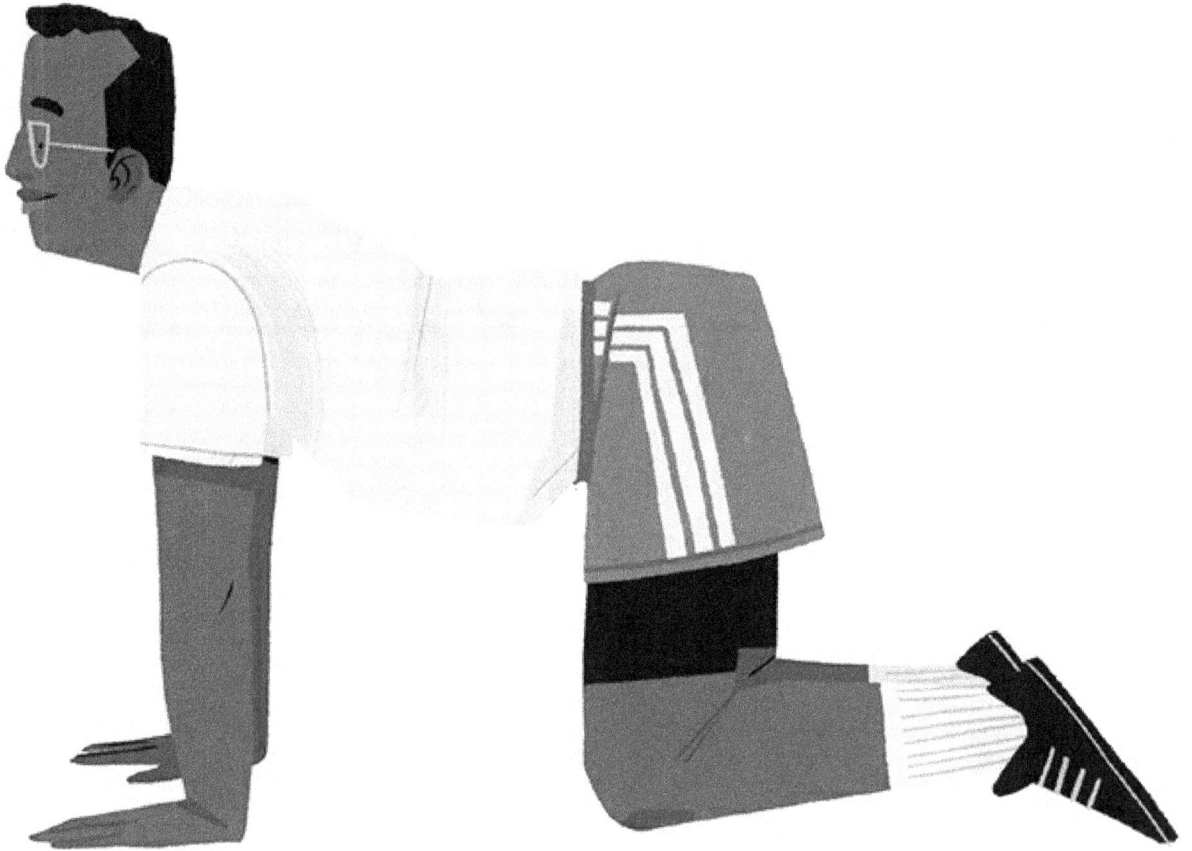

Cat Cow

Rectus abdominis　Transverse abdominis　Transversospinalis　Erector spinae

This seemingly easy move is an amazing pain reliever for lower back and sciatica pain. It strengthens and stretches the neck, shoulders, spine, and hips while gently massaging the internal organs of the belly, which feels great and is good for digestion.

INSTRUCTIONS

1　Begin on all fours with your palms directly beneath your shoulders, knees directly under your hips, straight spine. Direct your gaze straight down toward your mat.

2　As you inhale, drop your belly toward the mat and lift your chin to gaze up toward the ceiling. Draw your shoulders away from your ears and imagine lengthening your belly, like a puppy stretching after waking up from a nap. This is "cow."

3　As you exhale, draw your abs toward your spine and round your back toward the ceiling. Release your neck and allow your head to drop forward, but don't force your chin to your chest. This is "cat."

4　Move back and forth slowly between cow and cat anywhere from five to 10 times, being mindful of your breathing.

Modification: If your kneecaps hurt, double up your mat or place a folded blanket underneath your knees. If your wrists hurt, try resting your forearms on the mat instead of your palms.

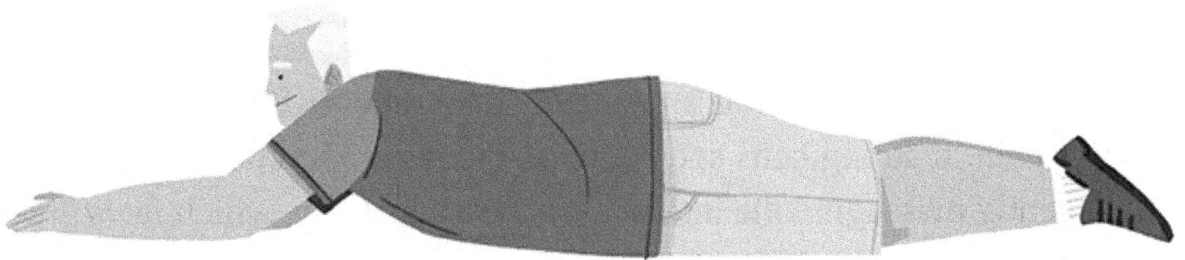

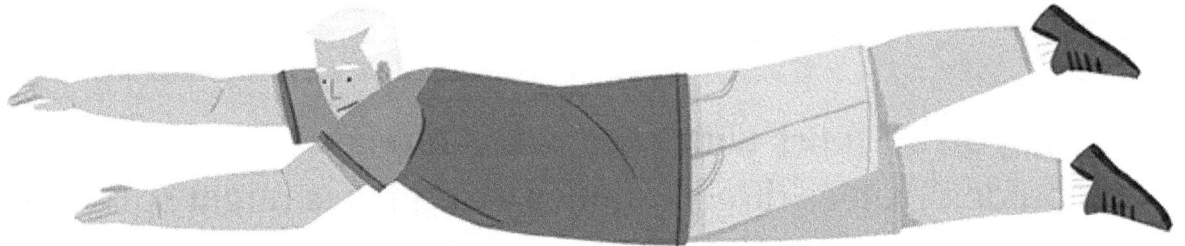

Alternating Superhero

Rectus abdominis / Transverse abdominis / Obliques / Erector spinae

Your core refers to more than just your abs. This exercise is great for targeting the set of muscles that wrap around your entire midsection, including the sides and back, which are essential for proper posture and for warding off that dreaded hunched spine as you age.

INSTRUCTIONS

1   Begin by lying face down on the mat, arms stretched overhead. Inhale.

2   As you exhale, raise your right arm and left leg a few inches off the ground, engaging your core to stabilize your body. Hold for 3 seconds, then release as you inhale.

3   Switch to the other side, raising the left arm and right leg off the ground, holding for 3 seconds. This is 1 rep. Aim for a set of 10 to 15 reps.

Modification: For an additional challenge, try increasing your tempo so your arms and legs make a "swimming" motion rather than holding at the top. Remember to keep breathing throughout.

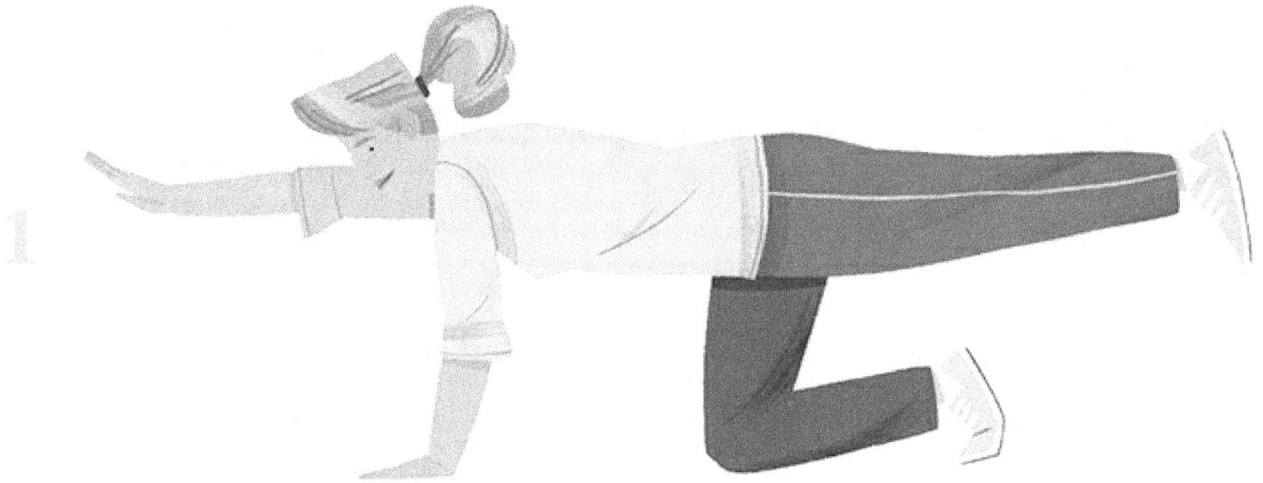

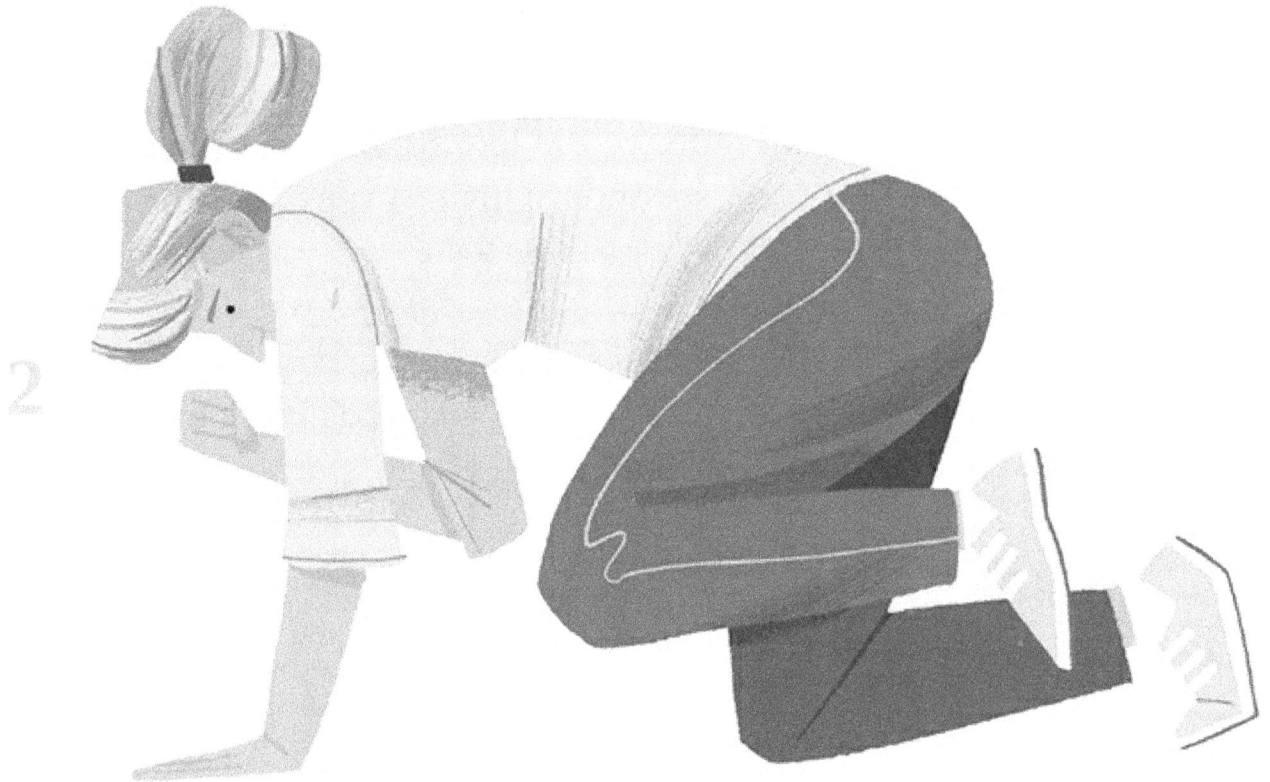

Bird Dog

TARGET MUSCLE GROUPS

Erector spinae / Rectus abdominis / Obliques

This exercise zeroes in on the muscles you need to safely extend, flex, and rotate the spine, which is key for independent movement. Bird Dog is a great exercise option if you're recovering from a back injury because it avoids putting pressure on the lower back.

INSTRUCTIONS

1. Begin on all fours with your palms under your shoulders and your knees directly under your hips. Gaze directly down toward the mat.

2. As you inhale, extend your right arm straight forward and your left leg straight behind you. Aim to create a straight line from your right fingertips, down your spine to your left toes.

3. As you exhale, engage your core, round your back and crunch your leg and arm in to meet in the middle. This is 1 rep. Do 10 to 12 reps, then repeat on the other side.

Modification: If you're having trouble balancing, try simply lifting your arm and leg a few inches off the mat and holding it for 2 to 3 seconds. Add the crunch later as you improve your balance.

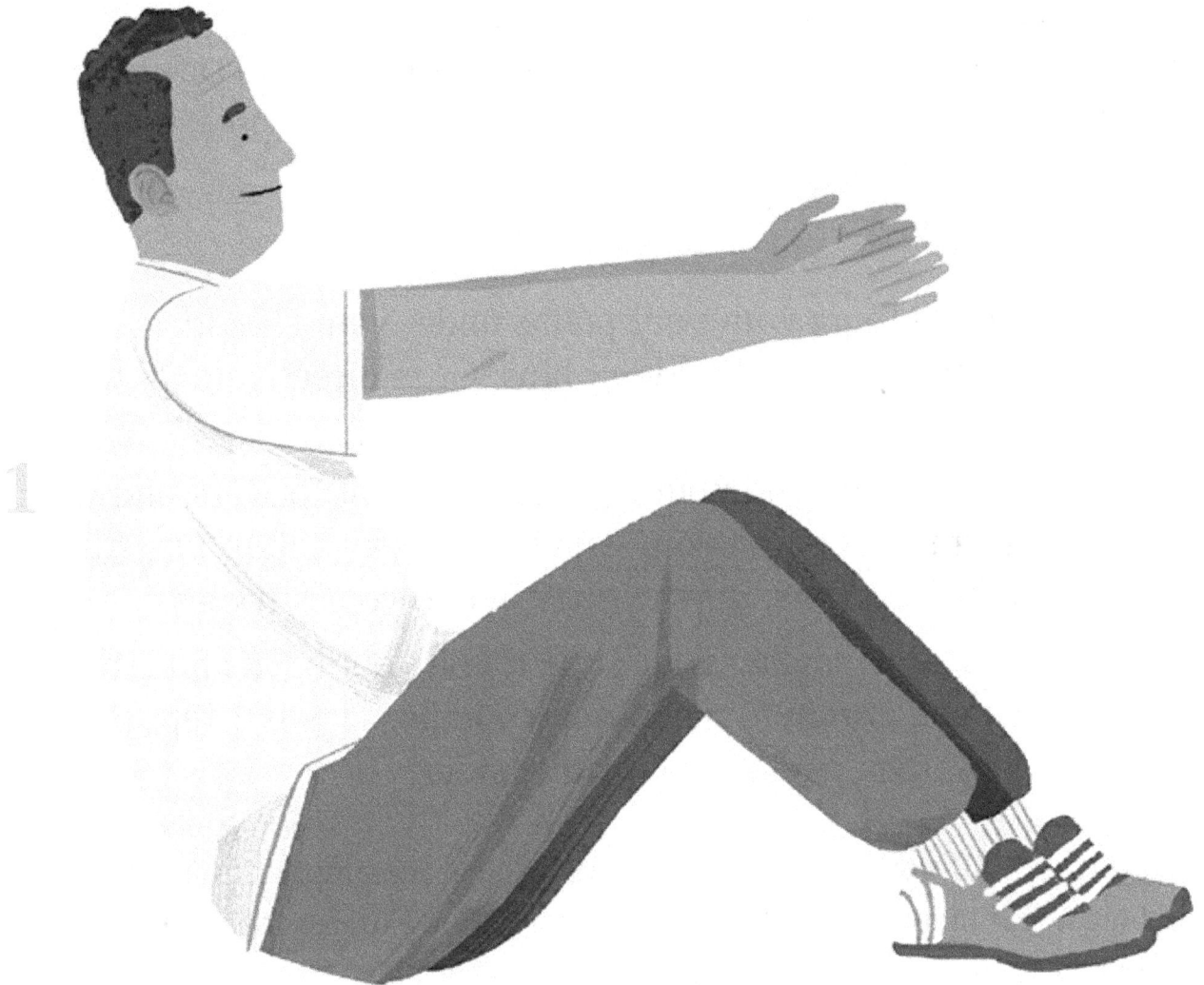

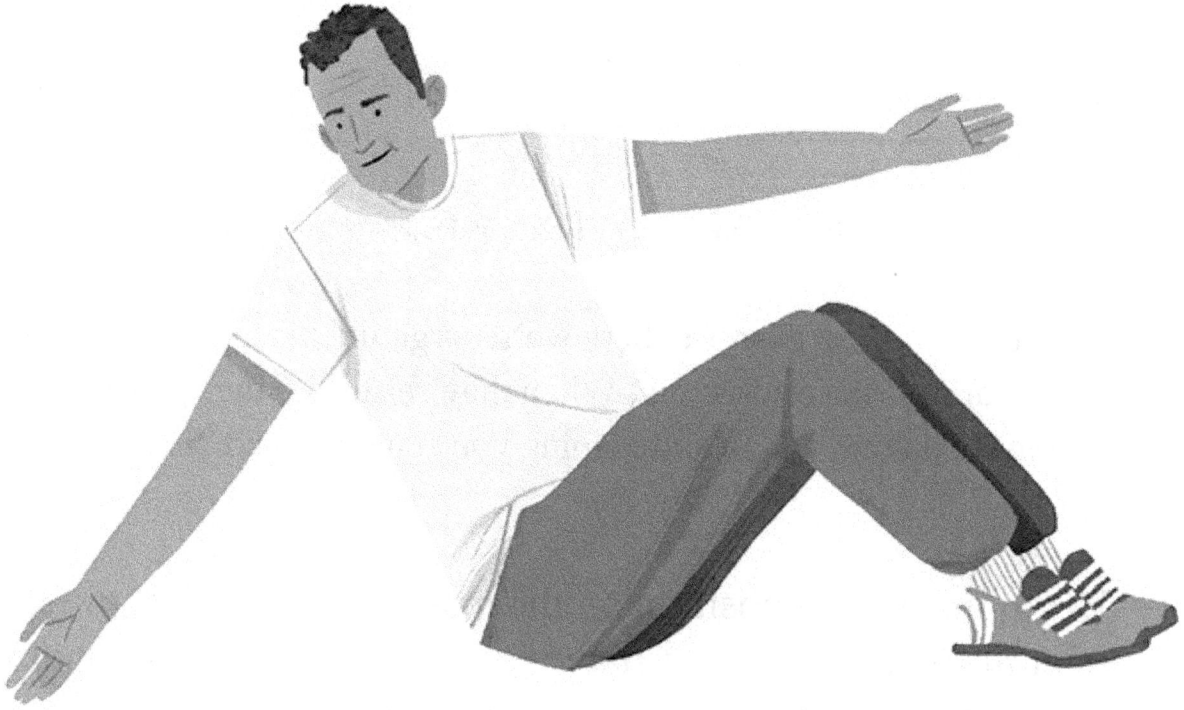

Side Sweeps

Transverse abdominis   Rectus abdominis   Obliques

Just as in the Bird Dog exercise, here we're targeting those muscles that wrap all the way around the midsection. When they're strong, they function like a natural girdle, pulling you in and helping you stand tall and move freely.

INSTRUCTIONS

1   Begin in a seated position on the mat with a straight spine, legs bent in front of you, feet flat on the mat. Reach your hands forward, keeping your arms about shoulder-width apart. Inhale.

2   As you exhale, rotate your torso to the right, sweeping your right arm out and around to touch the mat behind you.

3   Engage your core and inhale as you return to center. Repeat the sweep on the left side. This is 1 rep. Aim for 10 to 15 reps.

Modification: For less intensity, remove the arm sweep and perform the twist with your hands clasped in front of you or placed to the side of each hip on the mat.

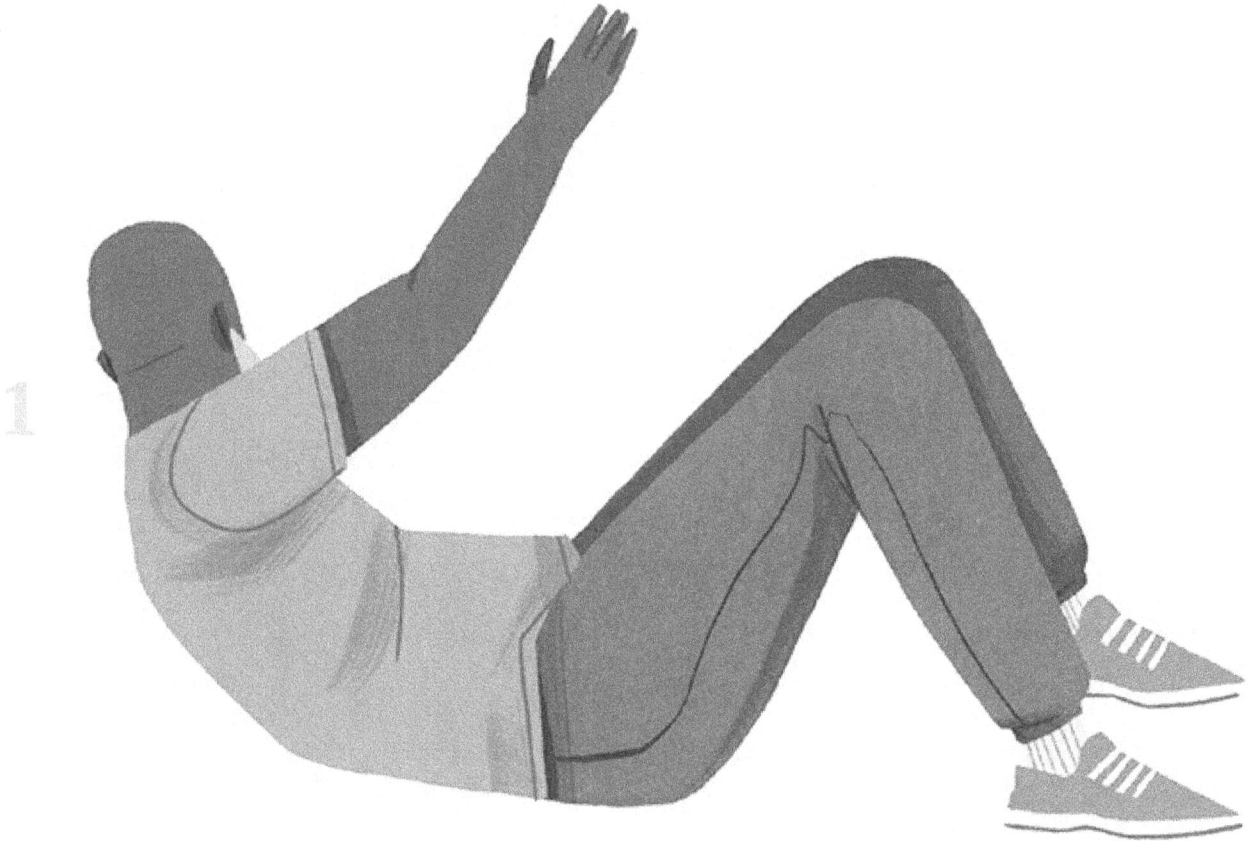

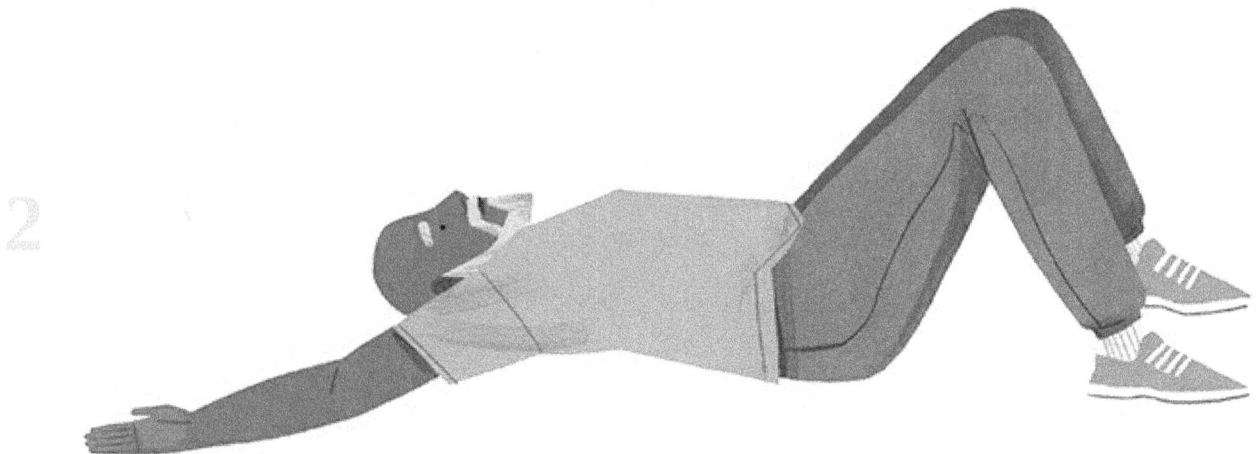

1

2

Lever Crunch

Rectus abdominis Transverse abdominis Obliques

Some people avoid getting down on the mat because they're not confident they'll be able to get back up again. But what happens if you fall? This exercise strengthens the muscles that will help you feel comfortable getting up from a lying down position, which is important not just in the case of a fall but also in the everyday activity of getting out of bed.

INSTRUCTIONS

1 Begin by lying flat on your back, legs bent in front of you, feet flat on the mat. Extend your right arm straight overhead and keep your left arm down by your side. Inhale.

2 Exhale as you contract your core and raise your right shoulder off the mat, sweeping your right arm up and over toward your left hip like a lever.

3 Inhale as you return to the starting position. This is 1 rep. Do 10 to 12 reps on each side.

Modification: Instead of returning to the starting position, remain up with your arm across your body and reach out toward the corner as in a pulse for 8 reps. Repeat on the opposite side.

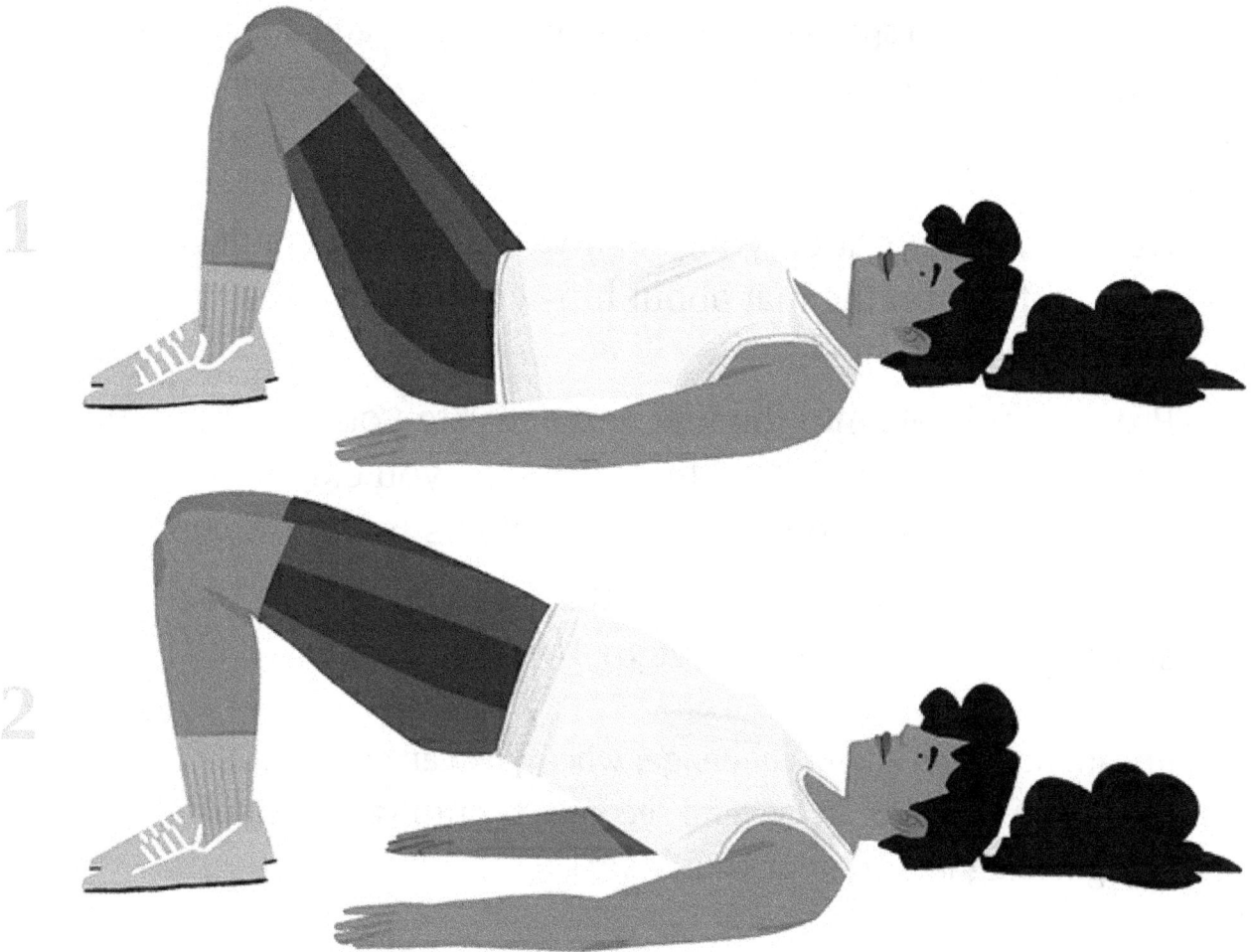

1

2

Bridge

Rectus abdominis / Transverse abdominis / Erector spinae

This is an excellent move for loosening up the muscles that get tight and constricted when you spend most of the day sitting. In addition to improving the range of motion in your hips, it'll help relieve hip and lower back pain.

INSTRUCTIONS

1 Begin by lying flat on your back with your legs bent in front of you, feet flat on the mat about hip-width apart. Rest your arms at your sides. Inhale.

2 Press your heels into the mat and activate your core and glutes, lifting your pelvis toward the ceiling as you exhale. Aim to create a straight line from your shoulders to your knees.

3 Hold for 3 to 5 seconds, then inhale as you release back to the starting position. Repeat five to 10 times.

Modification: For an added challenge, when you can comfortably hold the bridge with proper form for several seconds, try lifting one leg off the mat and straightening it in front of you.

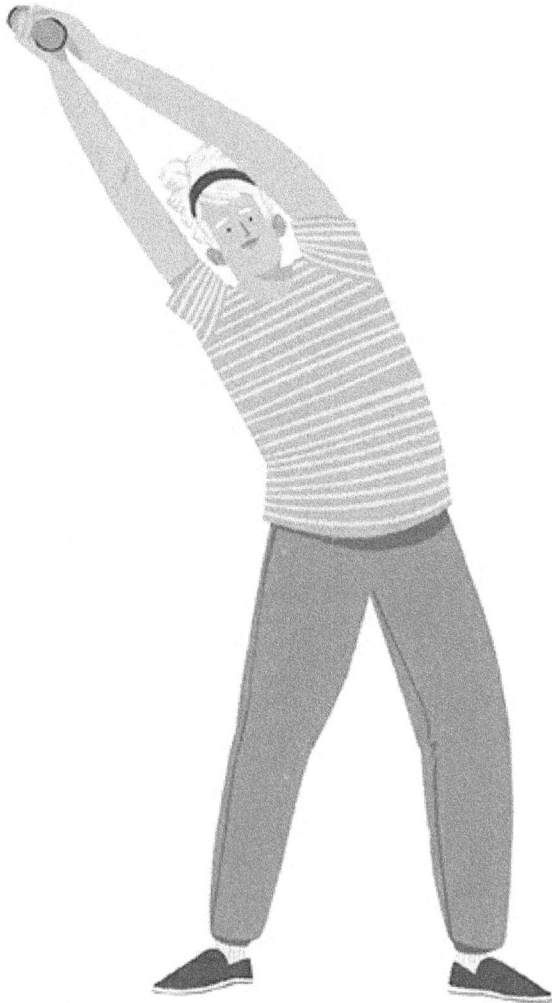

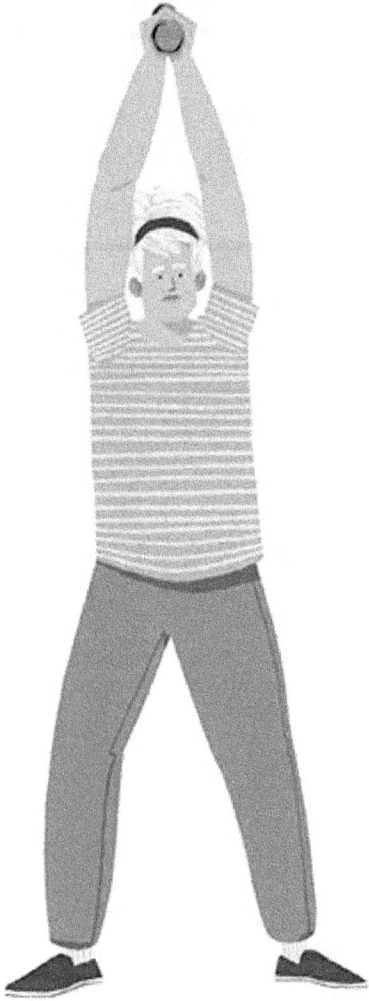

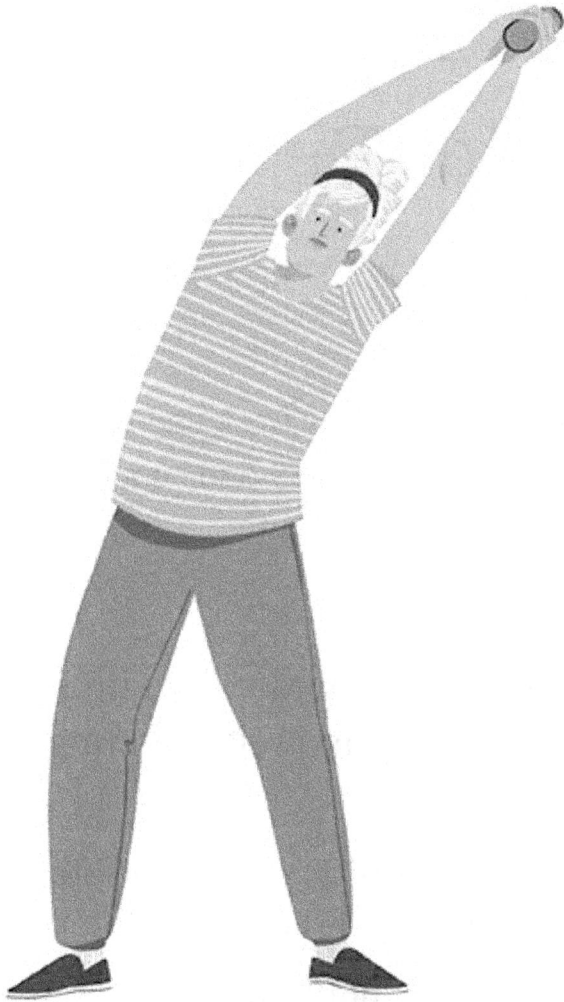

3

Dumbbell Side Bend

Obliques / Erector spinae

This move promotes strength and flexibility in the low back and the side abdominal wall, helping you move and bend more freely and supporting the spine. It also helps create definition in the waist.

INSTRUCTIONS

1   Begin by standing with your feet slightly wider than hip-width apart. Hold a dumbbell with both hands and raise it straight overhead. Inhale.

2   As you exhale, pull your abs toward your spine and imagine lengthening your spine as you bend slowly to the right.

3   Return to the upright position as you inhale, then repeat toward the left side. This is 1 rep. Aim for 10 to 15 reps.

Modification: If you need less intensity, practice doing the move with your hands on your hips before adding the dumbbell.

1

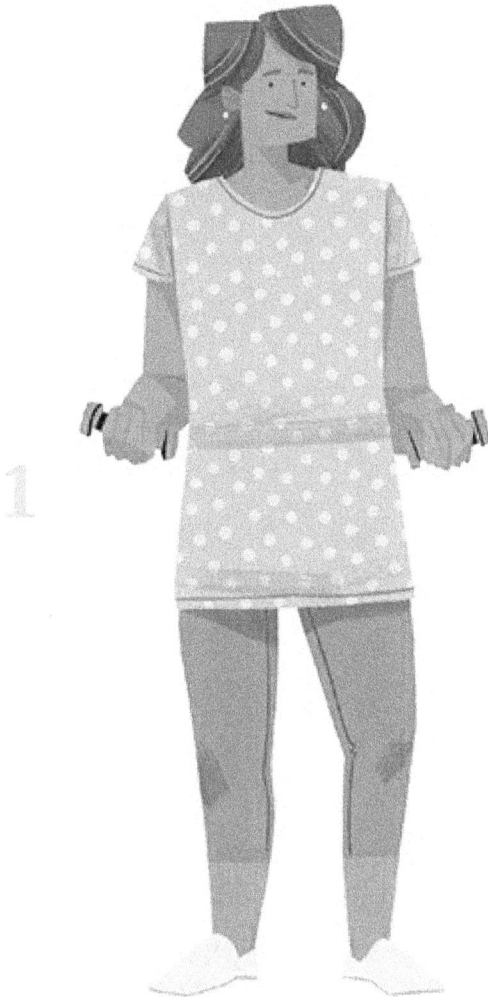

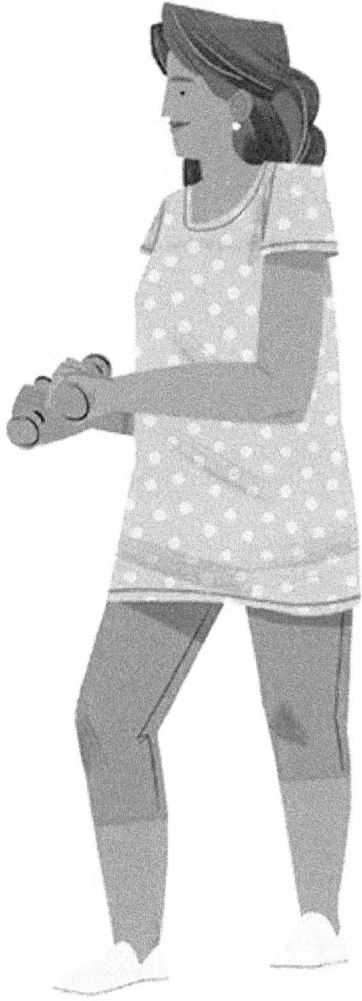

2

Twisting Lunge

TARGET MUSCLE GROUPS

Rectus abdominis Transverse abdominis Internal obliques

Rarely do you use only one muscle group at a time. Instead, you rely on multiple muscle groups from different parts of the body to work together successfully. Think of twisting to exit your vehicle and then rising to stand up. That's why moves that target multiple major muscle groups, such as this one that combines a side twist with a lunge, are such exceptional exercises to consider implementing into your life.

INSTRUCTIONS

1   Begin in a standing position, holding your weights at waist level, arms bent at a 90-degree angle, palms facing up. Inhale.

2   As you exhale, step forward into a lunge with your right leg, simultaneously twisting your torso to the right. Let your gaze follow the direction of your twist.

3   Inhale as you return to the starting position. This is 1 rep. Aim for 8 to 10 reps on each side.

Modification: For less intensity, try slowing down the move and breaking it into two parts—first the lunge, then the twist—rather than one steady movement.

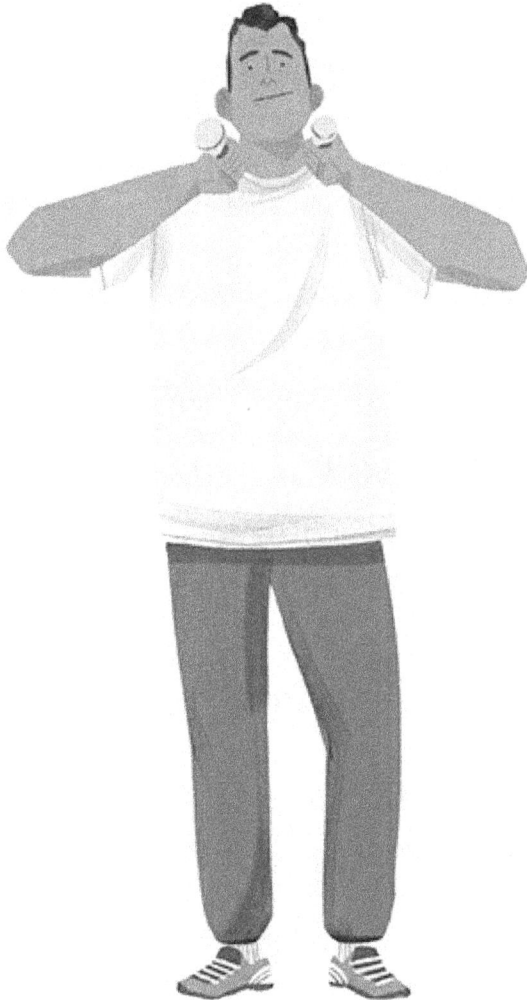

1

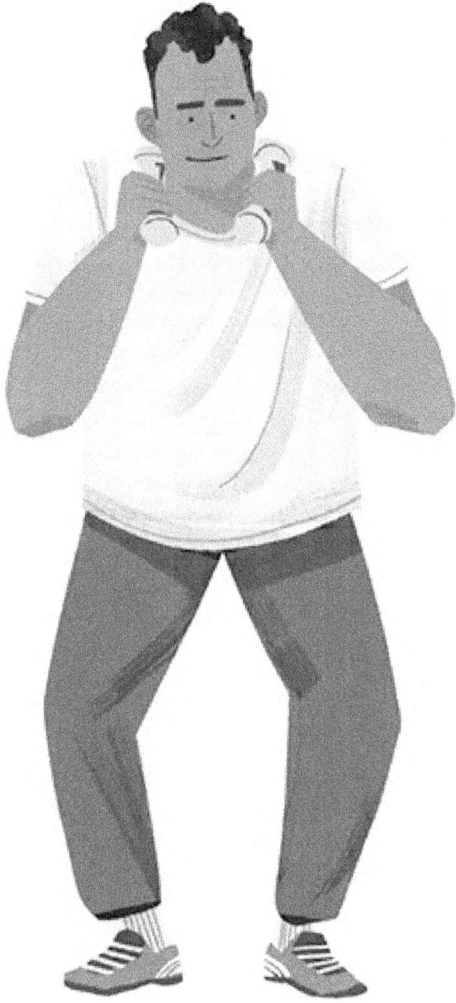

2

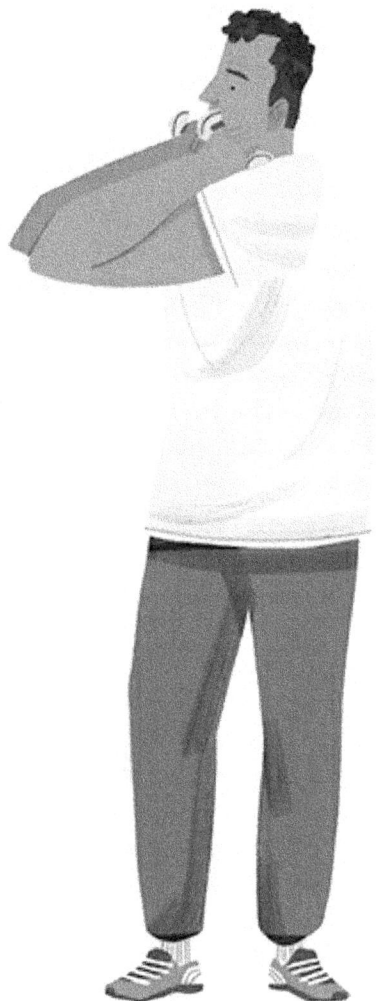

3

Squat with Twist

Rectus abdominis   Transverse abdominis

Incorporating squats into an exercise is a great way to up the calorie burn by engaging one of the largest muscle groups in your body. Practicing squats along with your core work will help keep you steady on your feet, along with improving your ability to bend and lift things as well as get in and out of a seated position.

INSTRUCTIONS

1   Begin in a standing position, feet slightly wider than hip-width apart, hands holding weights resting on your shoulders. Inhale.

2   As you exhale, send your hips backward and bend your knees, lowering as if preparing to sit in a chair. Avoid hunching forward; keep your chest upright.

3   As you inhale, press your weight into your heels to rise back to a standing position, twisting your torso to the right.

4   Repeat the move, this time twisting to the left at the top. This is 1 rep. Work your way up to 20 repetitions.

Modification: You don't have to squat super low for this exercise to be effective. For less intensity, don't sink as far into your squat, or perform the move without weights.

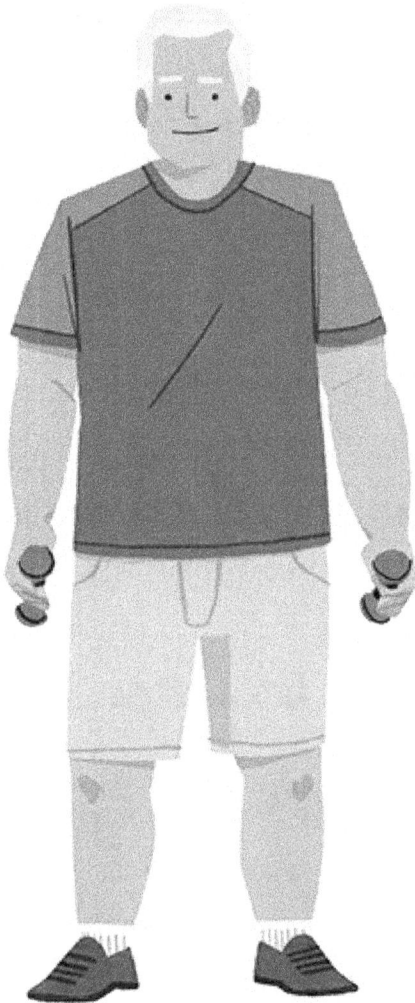

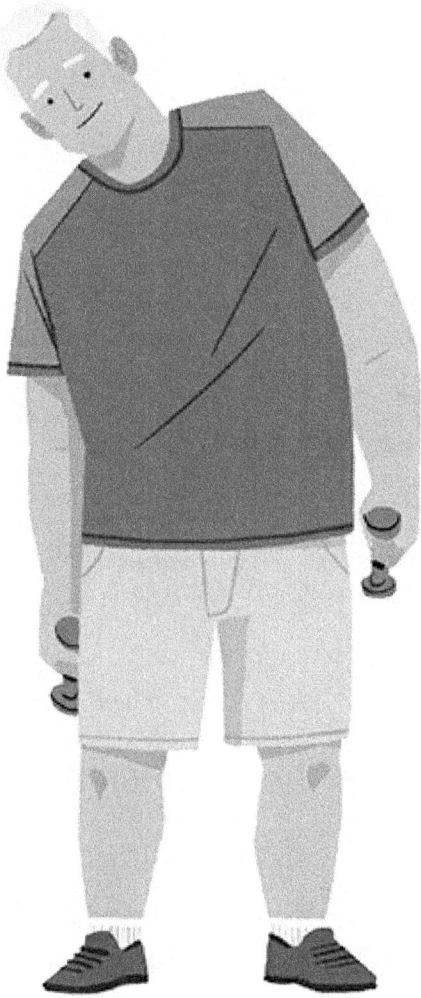

Reach Backs

Rectus abdominis   Transverse abdominis   Obliques

This exercise is a favorite for targeting the so-called "muffin top" that wants to hang over the top of your jeans. Reach Backs work the same muscles that assist in pulling your belly in, like an old-fashioned corset.

INSTRUCTIONS

1   Begin in a standing position with a dumbbell in each hand. Lift your chest and push your shoulders back and down, so your arms hang slightly behind your thighs. Inhale.

2   As you exhale, bend to the right, then to the left, reaching behind your knee on either side. This is 1 rep.

3   Continue breathing as you bend from side to side. Steady breathing is more important than when you inhale and exhale. Aim for 20 total reps.

Modification: For more intensity, increase the weight of your dumbbells, or perform additional reps several times in a row on either side and then reverse.

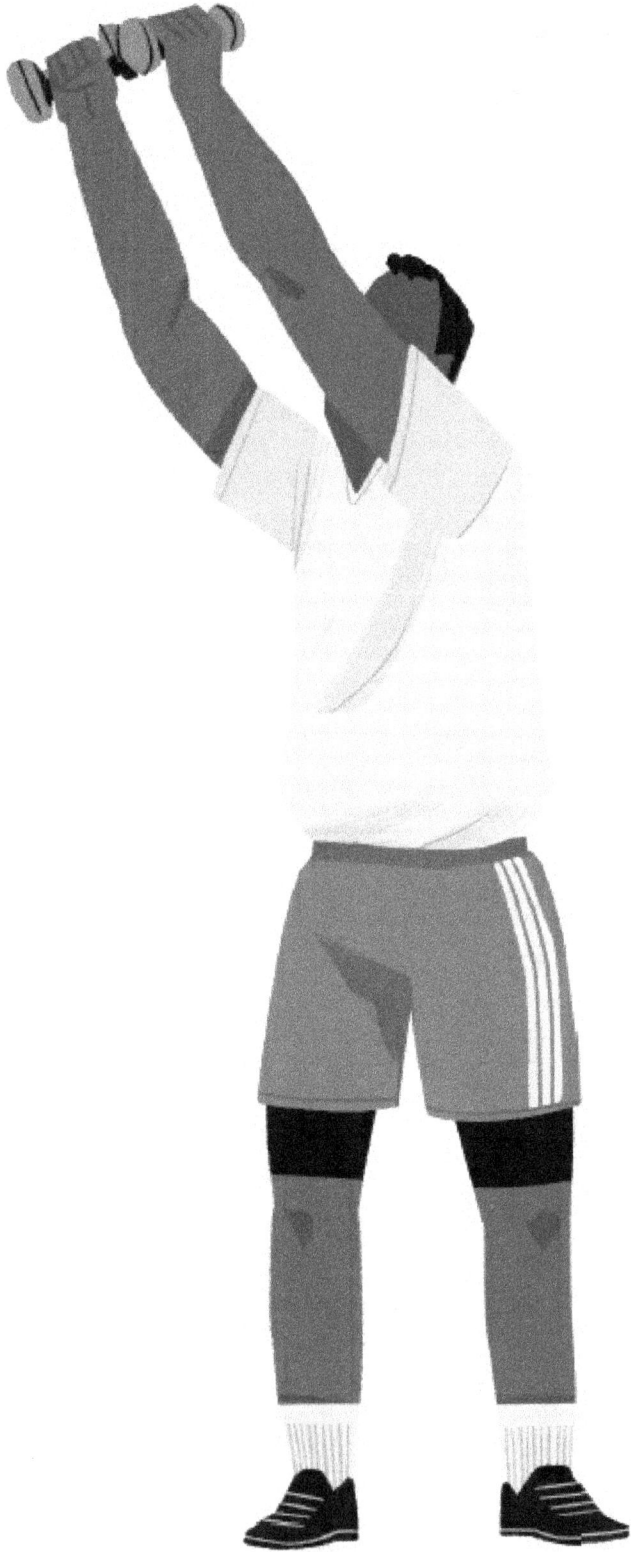

1

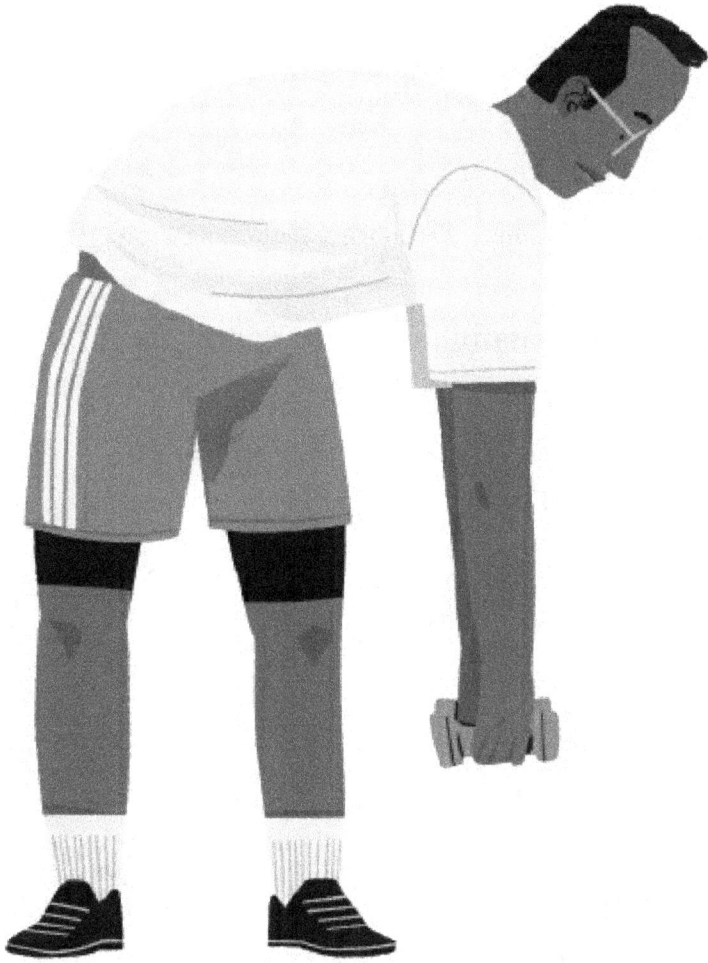

Weighted Pull-Downs

Rectus abdominis   Transverse abdominis   Obliques   Latissimus dorsi

This move strengthens the muscles and maintains the range of motion you need to safely perform a variety of activities. Putting away groceries, hanging decorations for a party, and trimming branches in your yard all activate these same muscle groups.

INSTRUCTIONS

1   Begin by standing upright, holding a dumbbell in each hand at chest level, arms bent.

2   As you inhale, reach up and to the right, shifting your weight onto your right foot.

3   As you exhale, engage your core and bring the weight down through center and across your body, squatting as you shift your weight to your left leg. Bring the weight to the outside of your left shin.

4   This is 1 rep. Perform 8 to 10 reps, then do the other side.

Modification: For more intensity, increase the weight of your dumbbells, or perform additional reps.

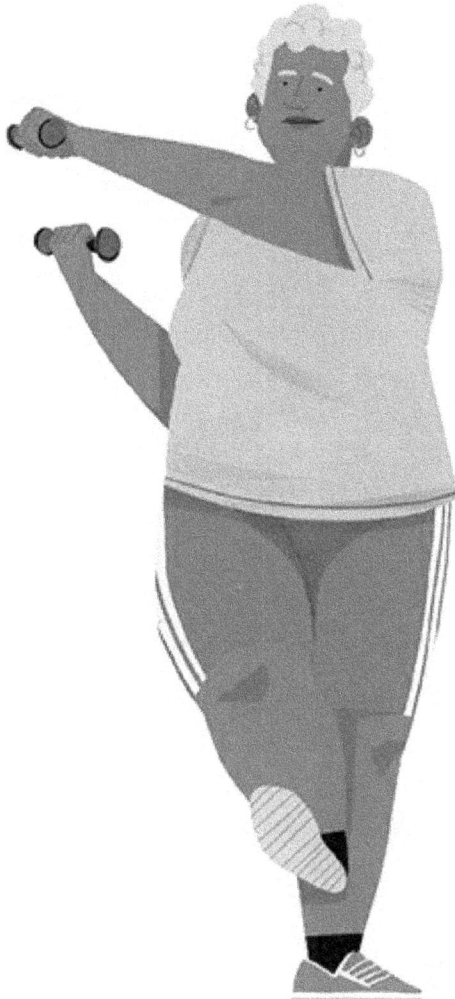

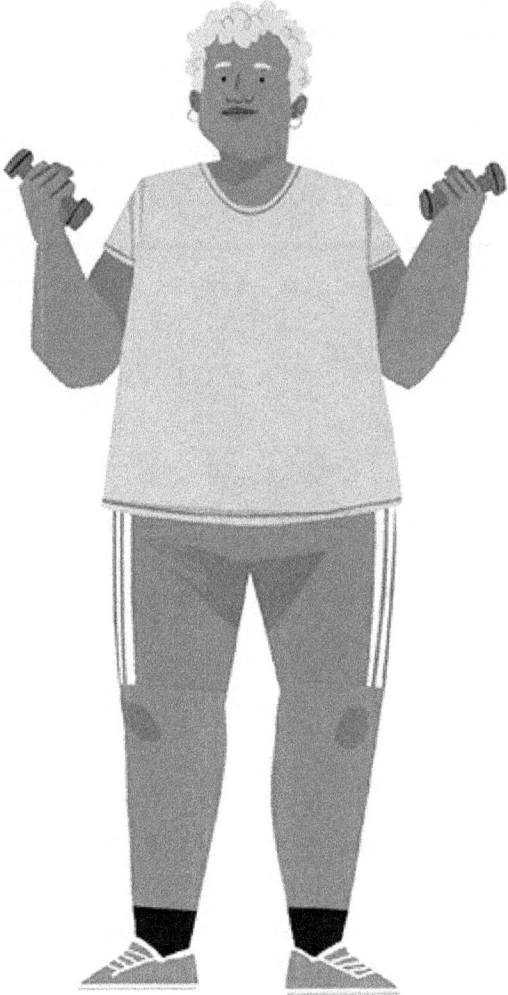

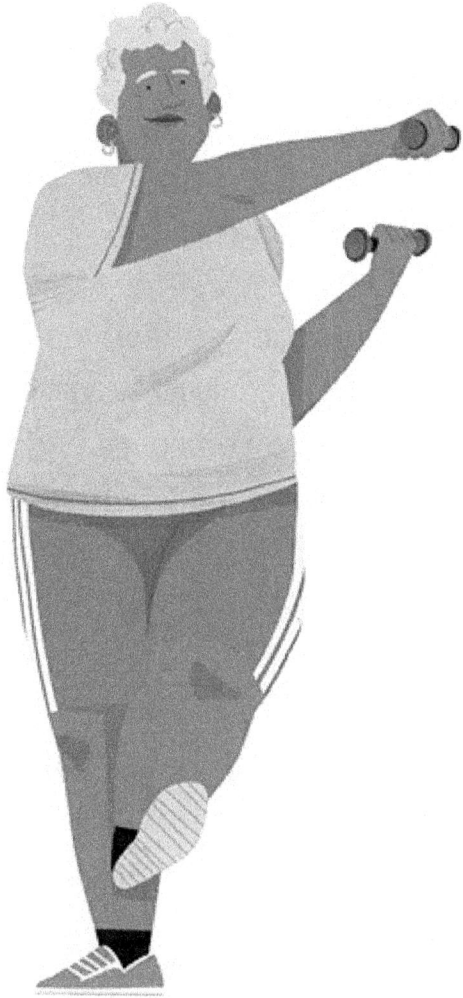

3

Punching Kicks

Rectus abdominis Transverse abdominis Latissimus dorsi

In day-to-day life, most of the time you're not thinking about how you move. Instead, you rely on your brain and muscles to work together to keep you balanced and upright. This move will work your balance and coordination, building muscle memory that will help you move safely even when you're not actively thinking about it. It also improves posture. For this exercise, a light weight is all you need. We often use one- or three-pound dumbbells.

INSTRUCTIONS

1   Begin in a standing position, a dumbbell in each hand, biceps curled. Inhale.

2   As you exhale, and with control, extend your right arm forward in a punching motion while simultaneously kicking your left leg forward.

3   Return to center and switch to a punch and kick on the other side, breathing steadily as you go. This is 1 rep. Aim to complete 20 reps.

Modification: Increase the weight or add reps for more intensity.

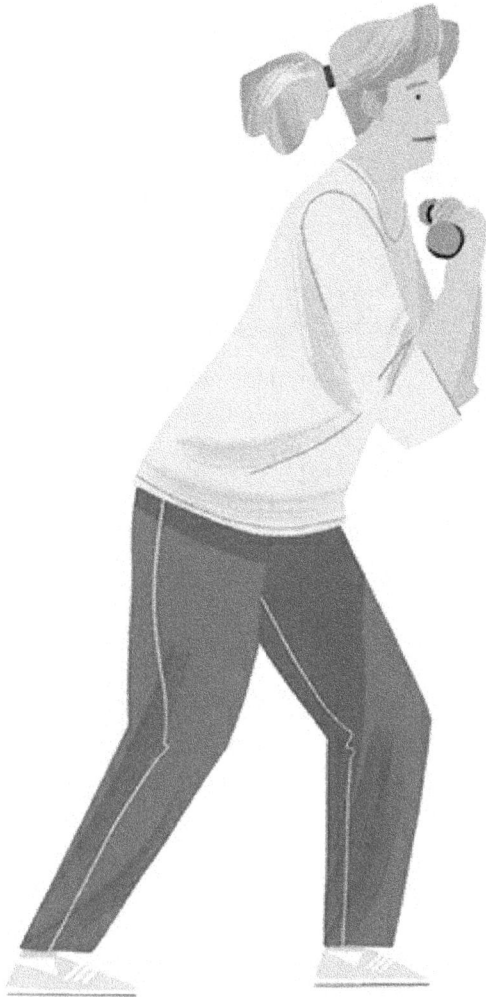

1

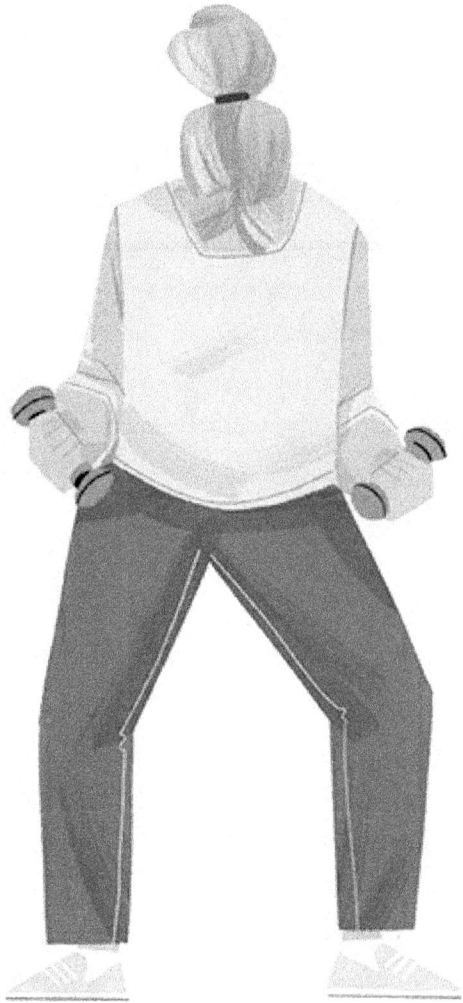

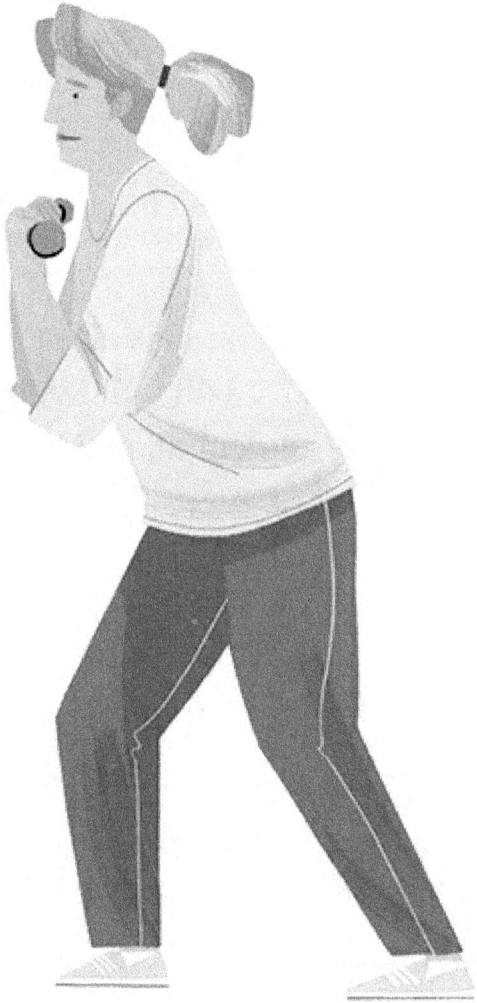

3

Crunching Twists

Rectus abdominis Transverse abdominis Obliques

In this exercise, you combine a squat with a twist; two great moves for building strength and toning targeted muscles. This move will build your ability to perform tasks closer to the ground, such as gardening, pulling weeds, or picking things up off the floor.

INSTRUCTIONS

1 Begin by facing to your right with your weight on your right foot, slight bend in the knees. Hold a dumbbell in each hand, biceps curled. Inhale.

2 As you exhale, engage your core and move to a squat position in the center, bending at the waist to bring your upper body into a crunch.

3 Inhale as you pivot to the left, lifting your torso to assume the standing position on the opposite side. This is 1 rep. Aim for 10 to 12 back-and-forth reps.

Modification: For more intensity, add an upward punch as you raise your torso to either side.

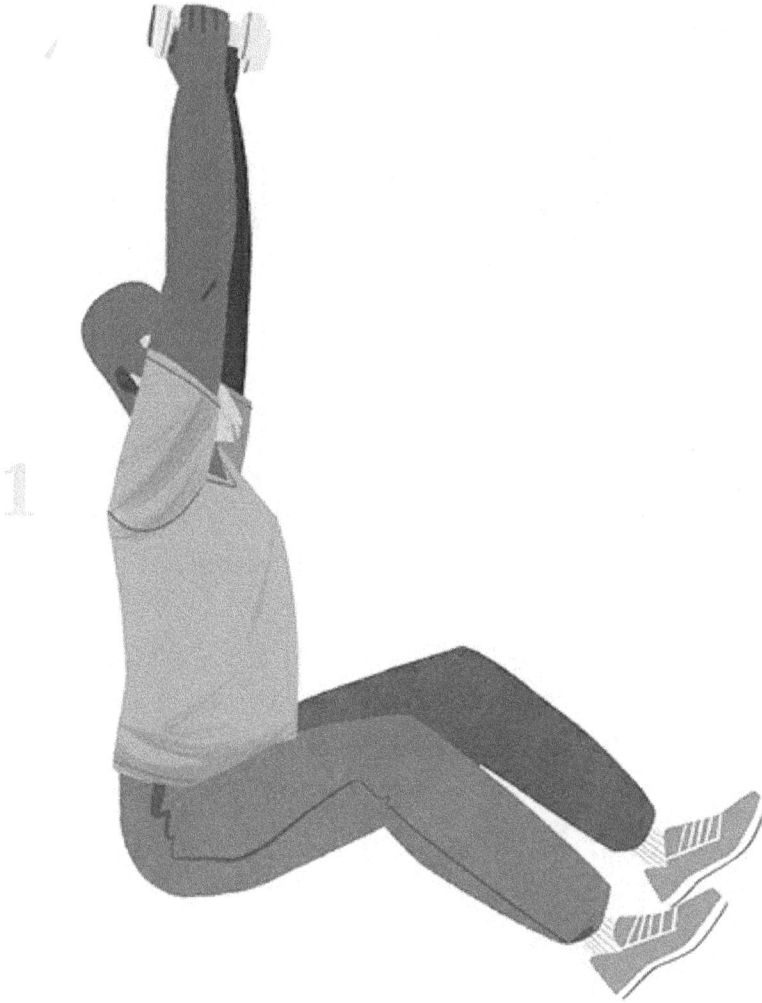

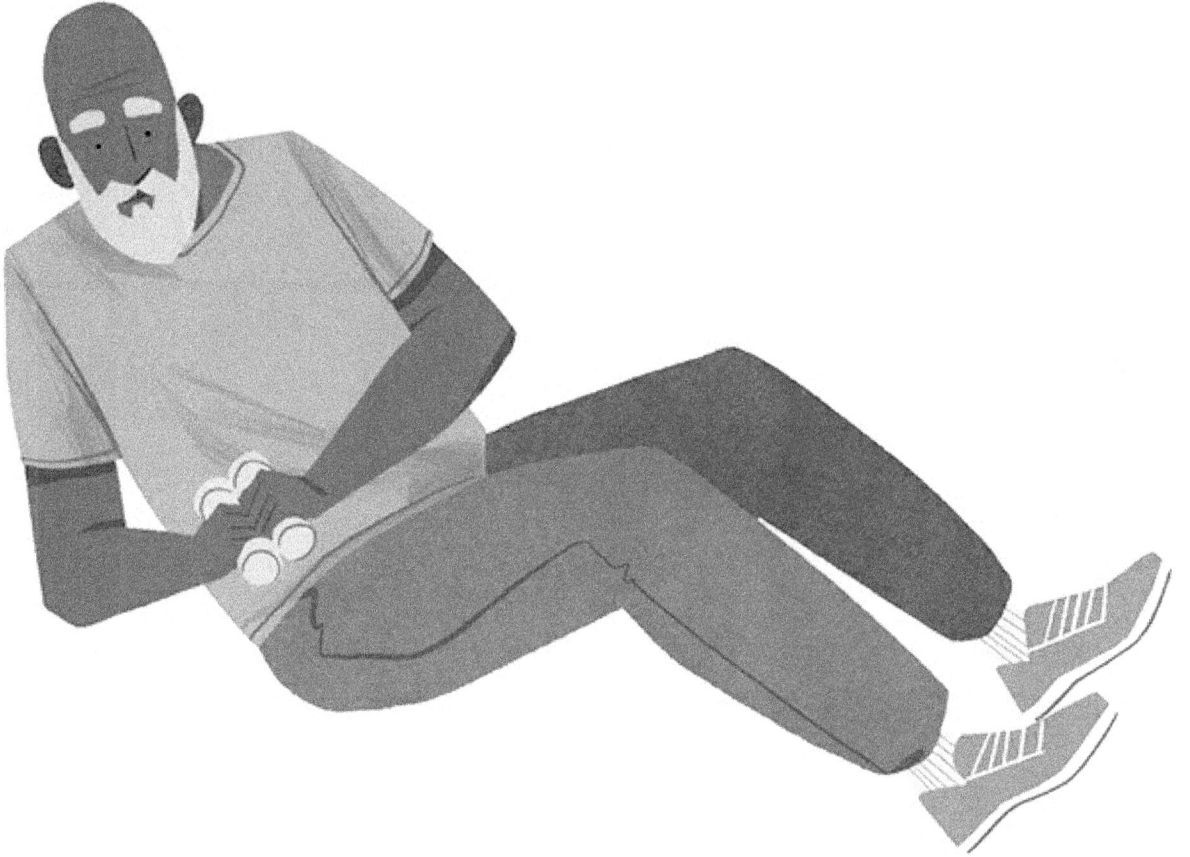

Angled Side Crunch

Rectus abdominis   Transverse abdominis   Obliques

This is a great move for building core stability as you challenge yourself not to wobble from side to side. It's a good one for keeping the muscles strong enough to help you roll sideways and lift yourself out of bed. Also, unlike traditional crunches, there's a much lower risk of injury to the neck while performing this move.

INSTRUCTIONS

1   Begin in a seated position on the mat, legs bent in front of you, feet on the mat. Hold one dumbbell in both hands and raise it straight overhead, sitting up tall. Inhale.

2   As you exhale, lean backward and twist your torso to the right, bringing the weight down and into your right hip.

3   Inhale as you return to the top. Repeat the crunch on the other side. This is 1 rep. Aim for 15 to 20 repetitions.

Modification: Extend your reach from the hip to the floor behind you, creating a longer range of motion.

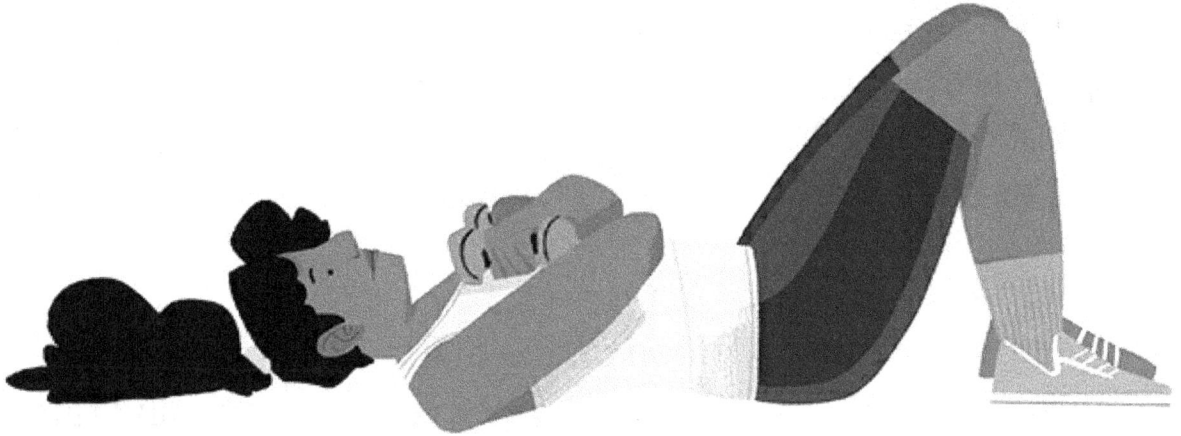

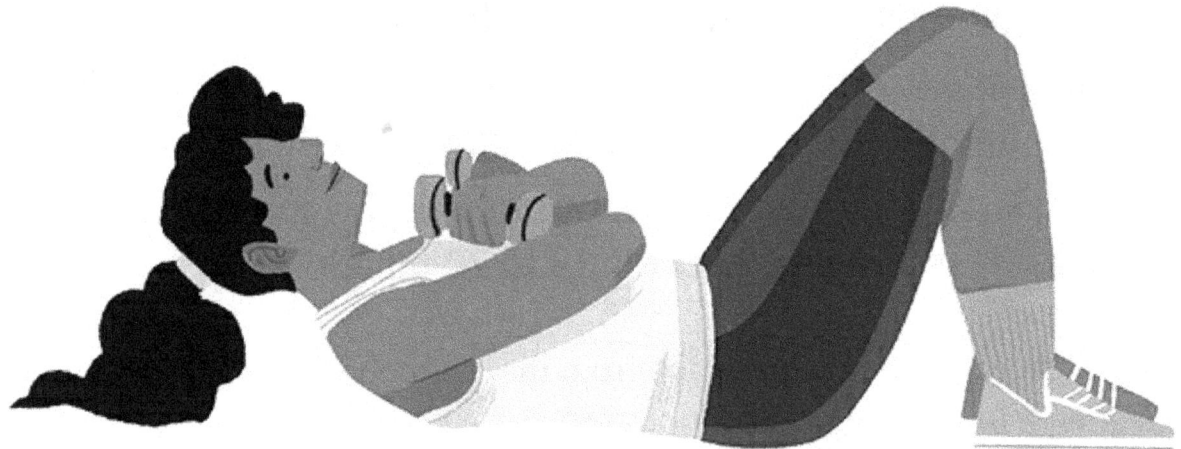

Weighted Crunch

Rectus abdominis / Transverse abdominis

This move is as close as we'll get to a traditional crunch in this book. The Weighted Crunch is an all-around good, low-impact exercise for building core strength.

INSTRUCTIONS

1   Begin by lying on your back, legs bent in front of you, feet on the mat. With a dumbbell in each hand, cross your arms in an X over your chest. Inhale.

2   As you exhale, engage your core and lift your chin toward the ceiling, bringing your shoulders off the mat.

3   Inhale as you lower your shoulders. This is 1 crunch. Aim for 15 to 20 crunches.

Modification: For more intensity, hold the crunch for 1 to 2 seconds at the top, or add additional weight.

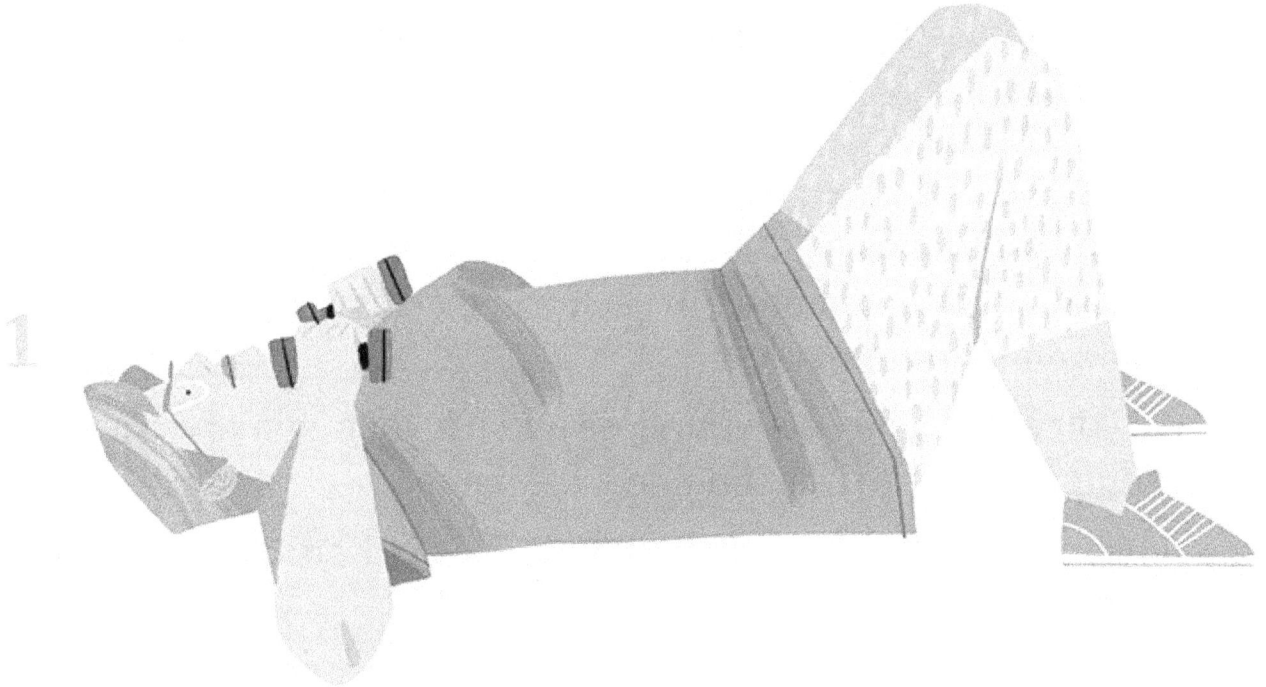

1

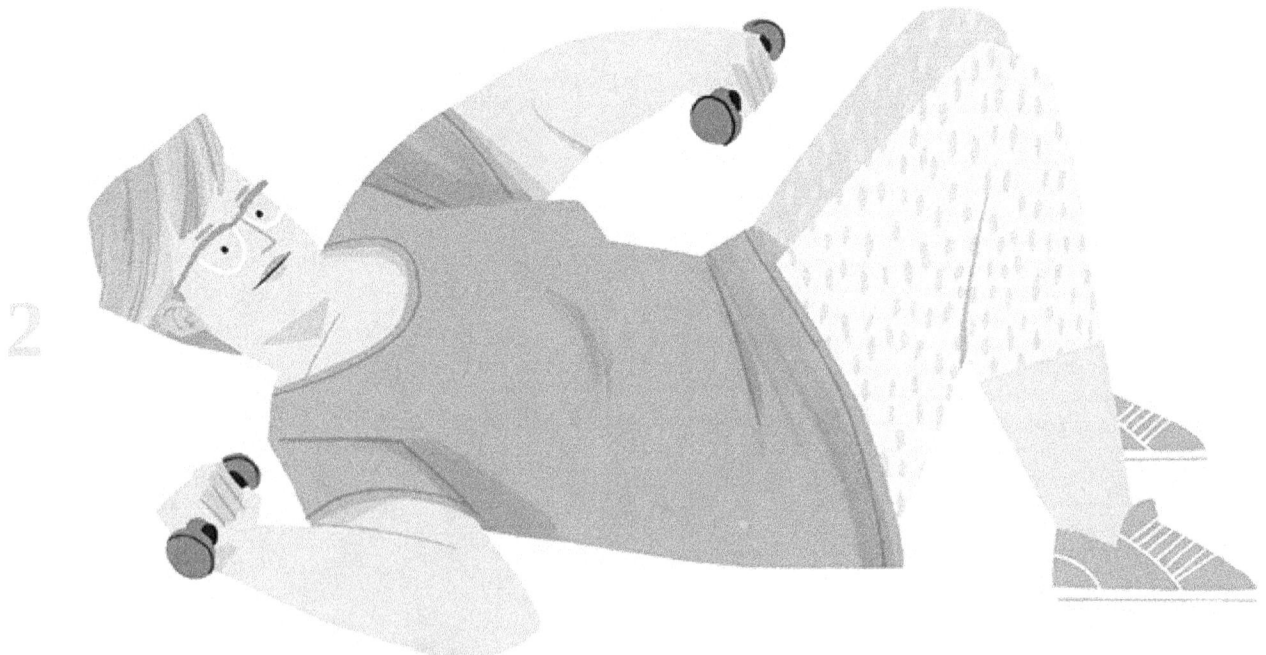

2

Punching Crunch

Rectus abdominis   Transverse abdominis

We love moves that do double duty, just like this one, which works the muscles of your chest while also firming your core.

INSTRUCTIONS

1   Begin by lying on your back, legs bent in front of you, feet on the mat. With a dumbbell in each hand, bend your arms and bring the weights to rest just above your armpits. Inhale.

2   As you exhale, engage your core and lift your shoulders off the mat, twisting your torso toward the right. Extend your left arm upward in a punching motion.

3   Inhale as you lower your back to the mat and return to the starting position. Repeat on the opposite side. This is 1 crunch. Aim for 15 to 20 crunches.

Modification: For more intensity, hold the punch for 1 to 2 seconds at the top, or add additional weight.

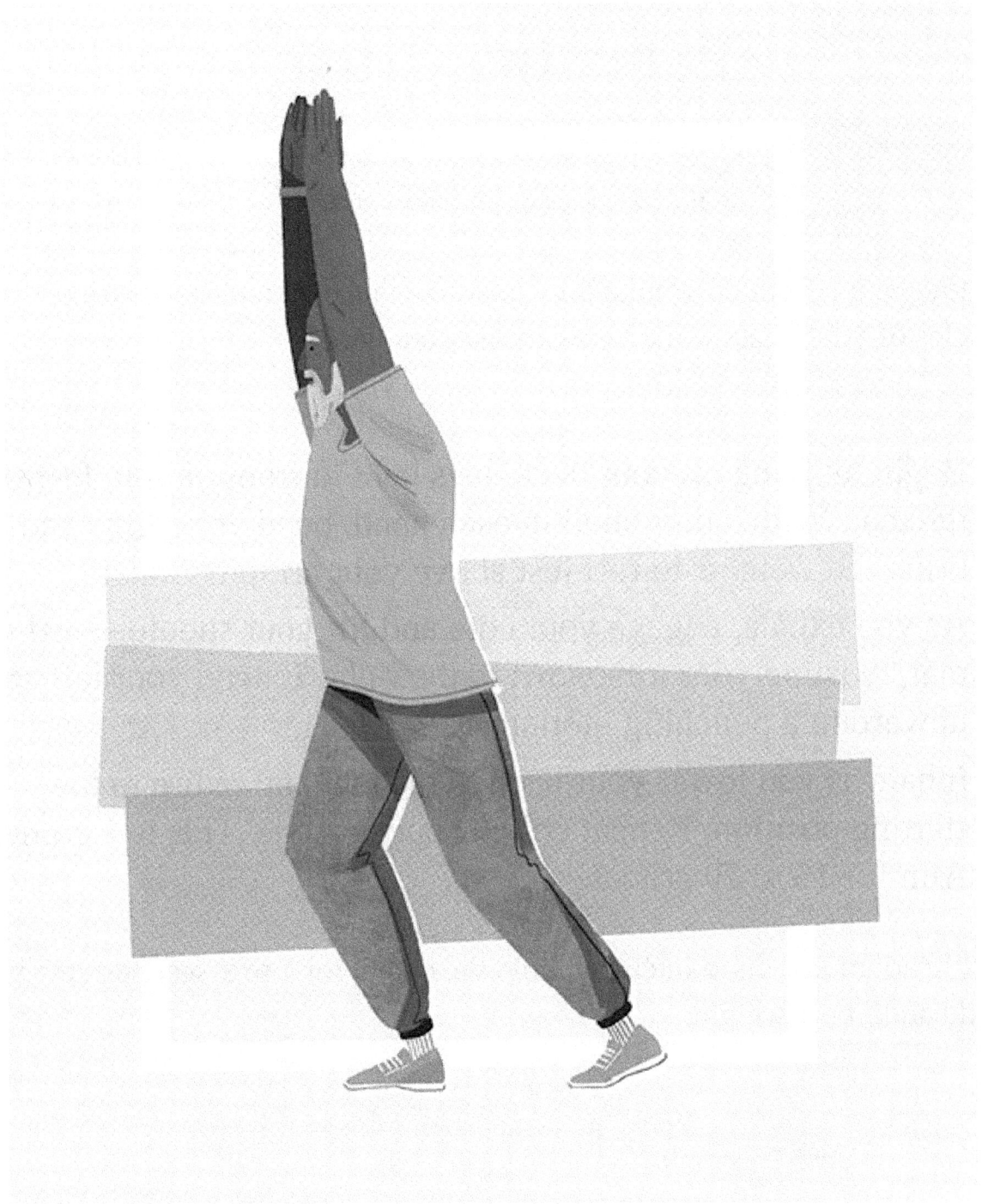

CHAPTER THREE

The Routines
Putting It All Together

Although you can certainly do any of the exercises from chapter 2 on their own, the following 5-minute workouts are meant to help you get even more mileage out of the moves. Together, they're more than the sum of their parts and each routine here ensures that you hit every major core muscle group. Each 5-minute routine is labeled with one of the following categories to help you select routines that will fit best with your needs.

Routines for Around the House. These routines will help you build stability for moving safely and comfortably through the motions of daily life in and around your house.

Routines for Active Living. These routines will help you stay mobile so you can be active with confidence in whatever activities you choose to pursue.

Routines for Aches and Pains. Like a machine, our bodies *need* motion to "grease the wheels" and keep the parts moving smoothly. These routines promote circulation that fights inflammation while building muscle mass to support strong bones.

Routines to Do with a Partner. Some things are more fun with a friend! Grab a buddy, family member, or spouse and pair up for these routines, which are easiest with a little extra encouragement or an extra eye to check your form.

Got five minutes? Great! Let's get started.

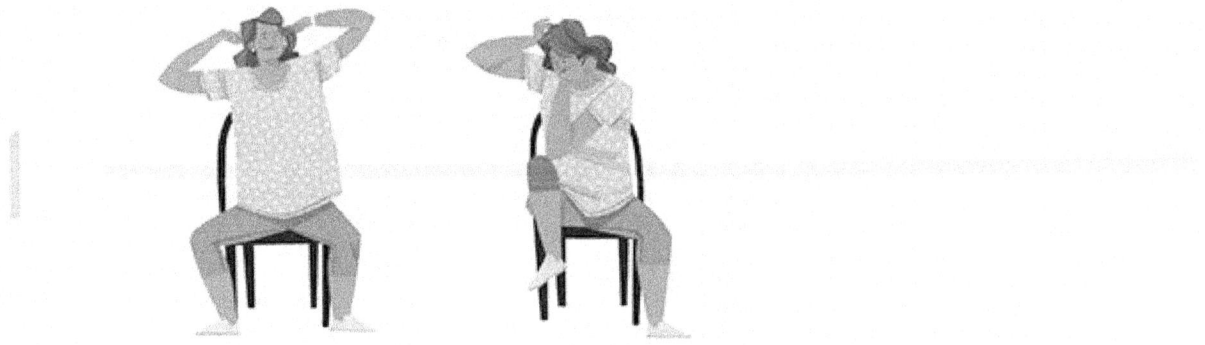

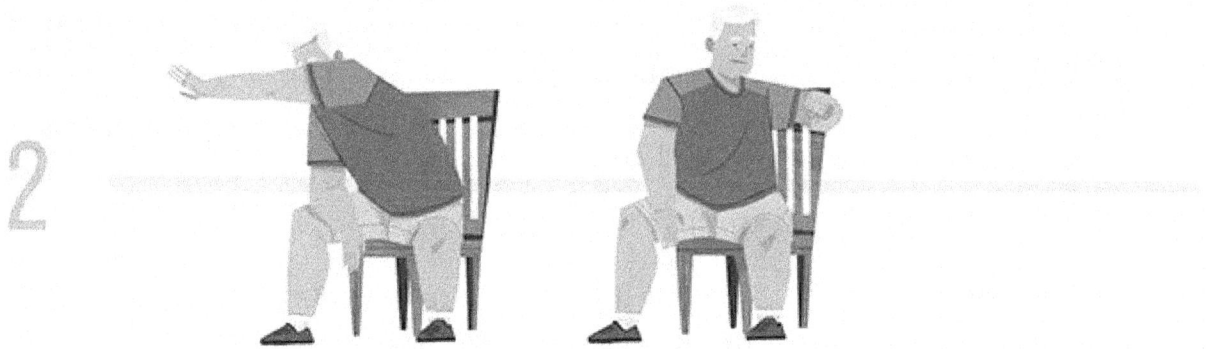

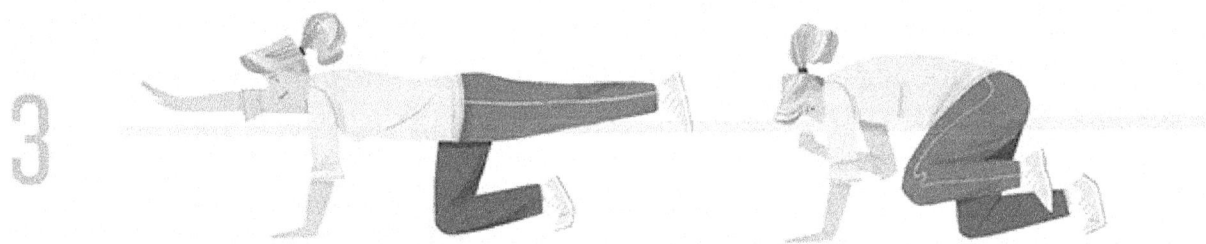

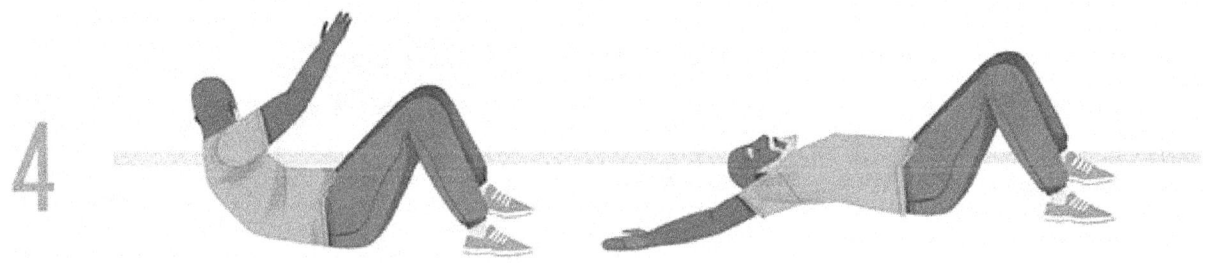

Spring Cleaning

ROUTINES FOR AROUND THE HOUSE

From scrubbing floors, to washing windows, to doing laundry, this routine will help you move comfortably and maintain your footing as you clean up around the house.

THE ROUTINE

1. Diagonal Crunch: 20 reps
2. Rope Pulls: 8 reps on each side
3. Bird Dog: 8 reps on each side
4. Lever Crunch: 8 reps on each side

Remember: Be mindful of your spine. During each of the exercises, imagine keeping a straight line from the crown of your head to the tip of your tailbone.

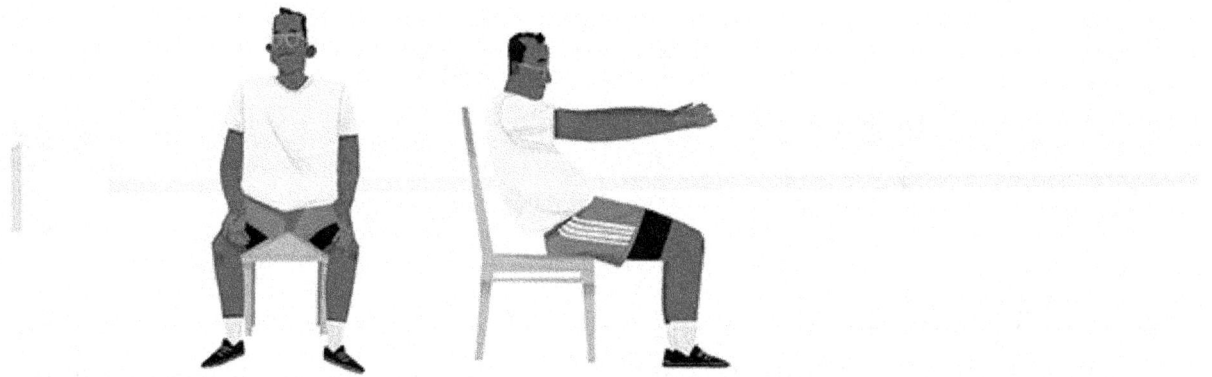

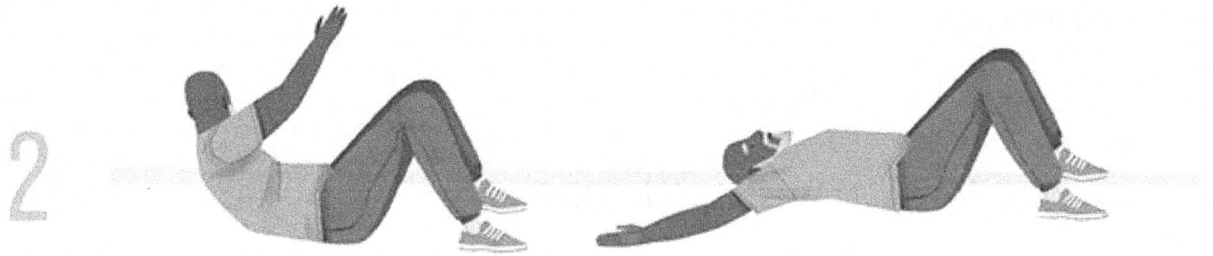

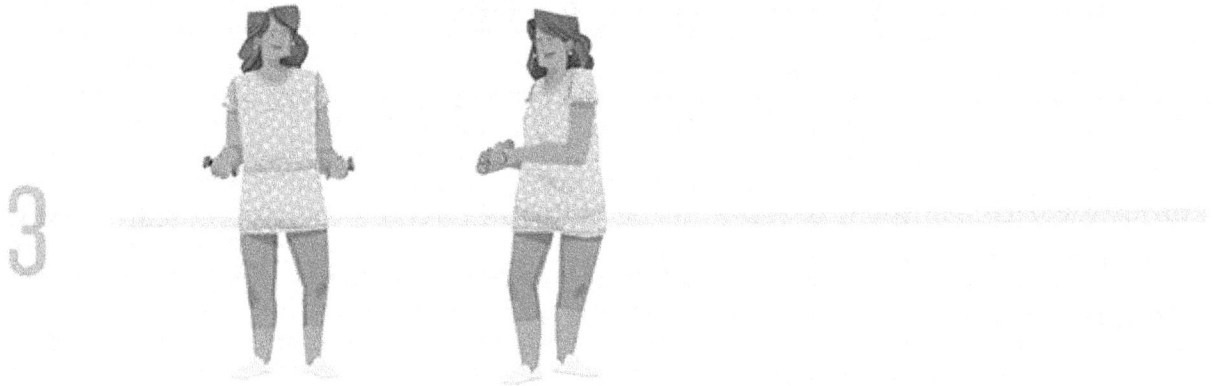

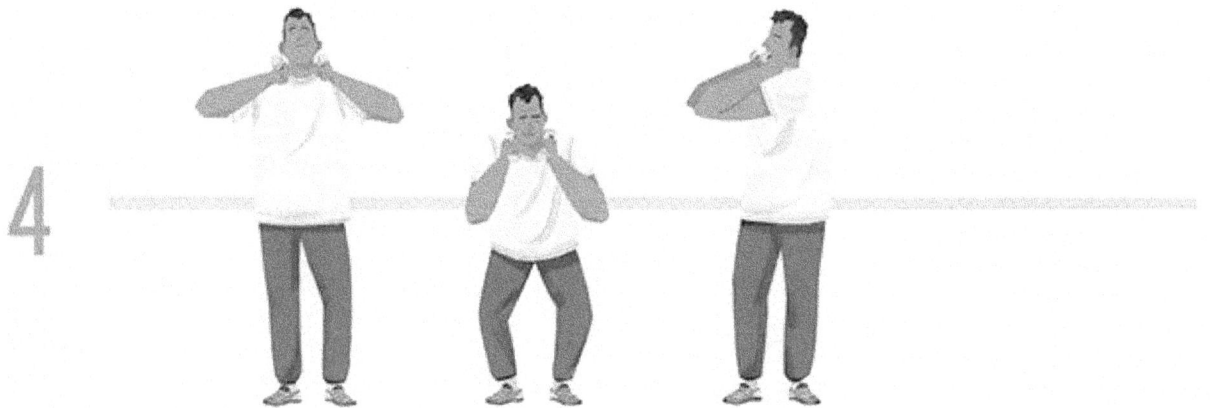

Up and at 'Em

ROUTINES FOR AROUND THE HOUSE

Does it take you a few tries to get out of your favorite chair? This routine will help keep you from getting stuck on the couch or in your recliner.

THE ROUTINE

1 Slow Recline: **10 reps**

2 Lever Crunch: **8 reps on each side**

3 Twisting Lunge: **8 reps on each side**

4 Squat with Twist: **20 reps**

Remember: Proper form is important to protect your knees during the Twisting Lunge and Squat with Twist. Really sink down into the squat and lunge position, keeping the bulk of your weight in your heels rather than allowing your heels to come off the ground.

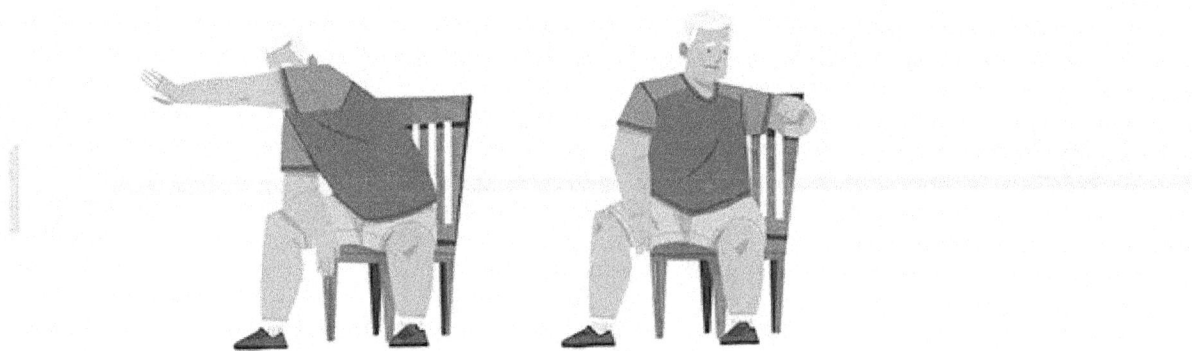

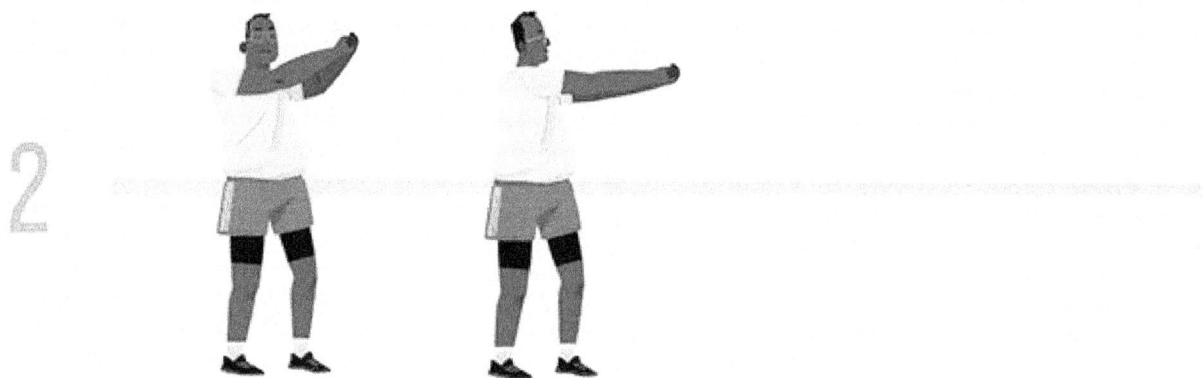

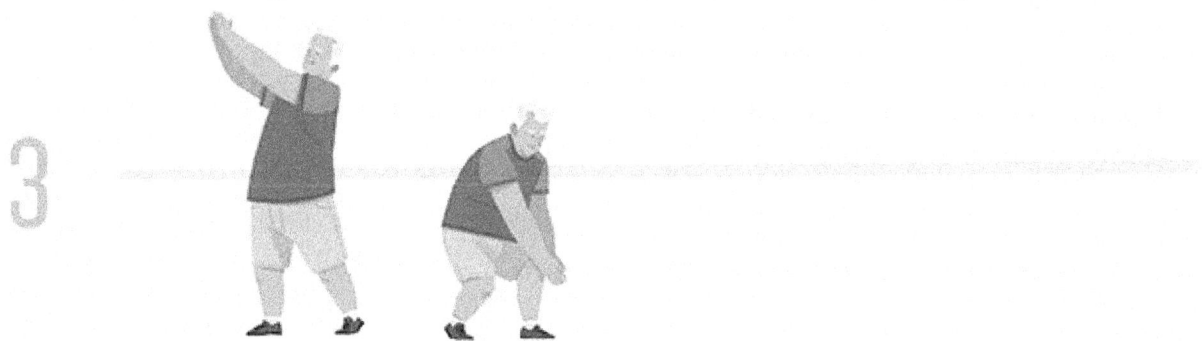

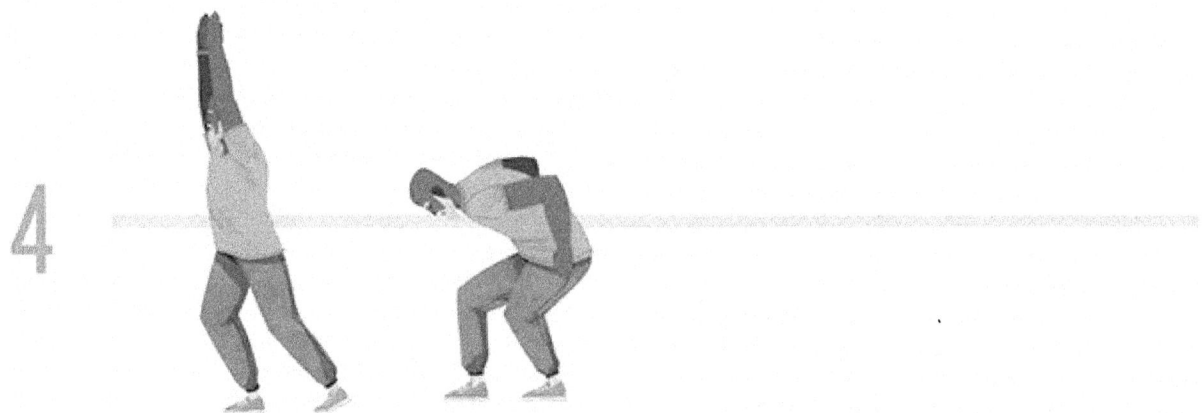

What's Cooking

ROUTINES FOR AROUND THE HOUSE

This routine will help you maintain the wide range of motion used in kitchen activities, such as pulling ingredients off a shelf, grabbing something from a low cabinet, twisting to reach for a utensil, or unloading the dishwasher.

THE ROUTINE

1 **Rope Pulls**: 8 reps on each side

2 **Torso Twists**: 8 reps

3 **Wood Chop**: 8 reps on each side

4 **Diagonal Sit Back**: 8 reps on each side

Remember: Let your core do the majority of the work rather than using the momentum from your arm motions to accomplish the move. You can check yourself on this by doing one or two reps without the arms.

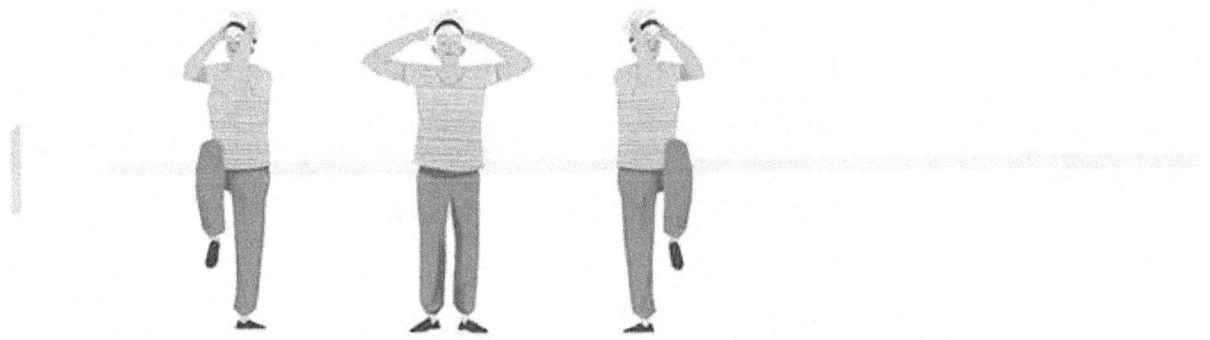

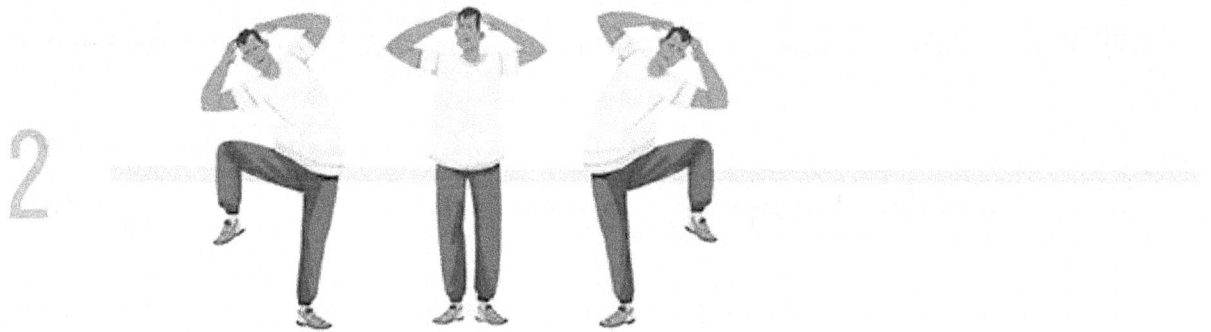

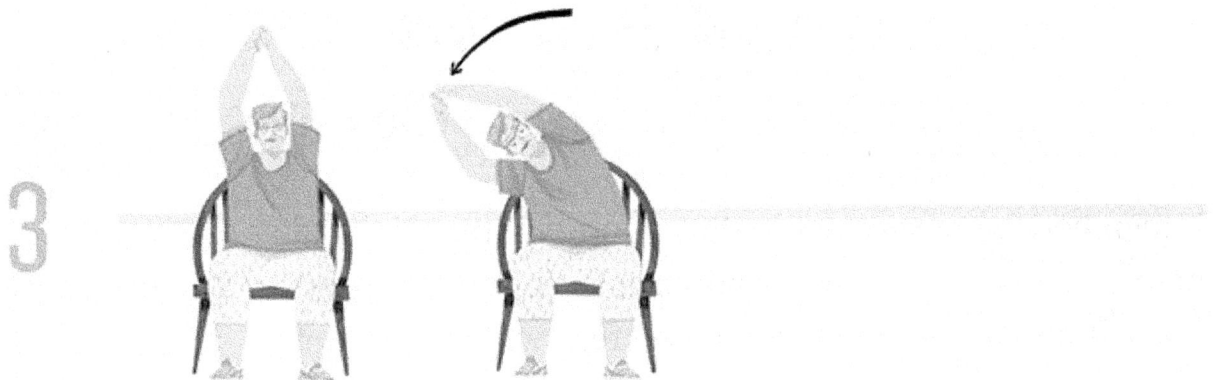

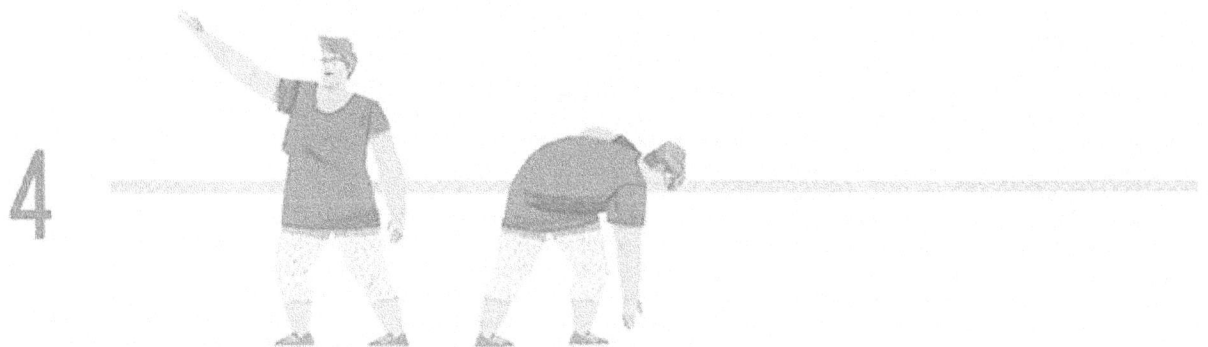

Strong and Steady

ROUTINES FOR AROUND THE HOUSE

One in four people older than 65 experience a fall each year, and the majority of those falls happen in the home. This routine builds the stability you need to have "successful" falls . . . and prevent them happening in the first place.

THE ROUTINE

1   Standing Crunch: 20 reps

2   Side Crunch with Leg Lift: 8 reps on each side

3   Metronome: two 30-second cycles with a short break between cycles

4   Cross Pull-Down: 8 reps on each side

Remember: When you're working on balance, where you focus your vision matters. Try to avoid looking down at the floor; instead, keep your chin lifted and direct your gaze toward a focal point in front of you.

1

2

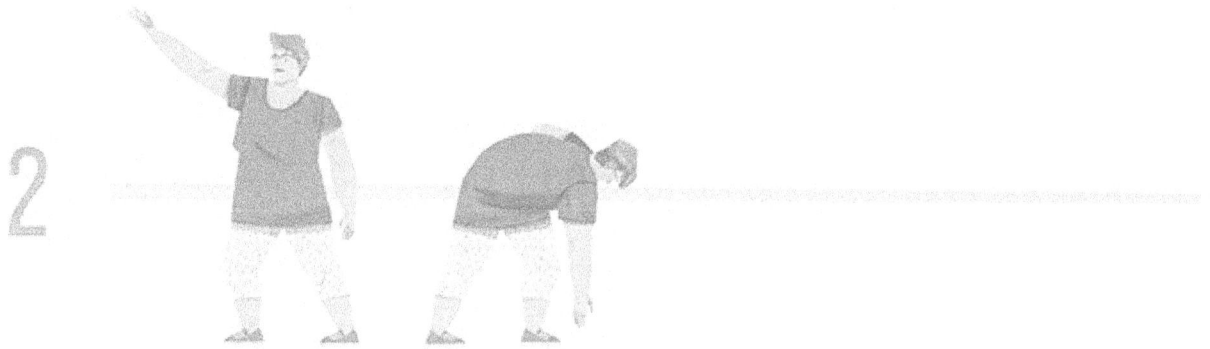

3

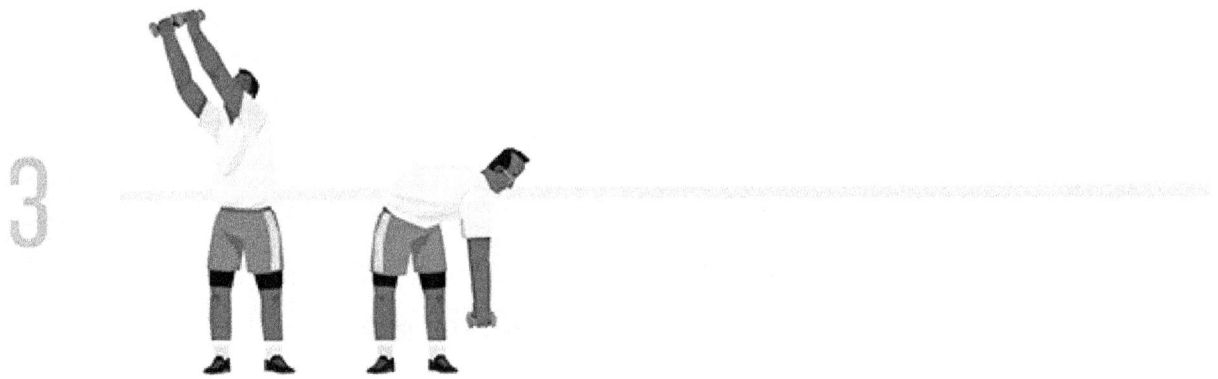

4

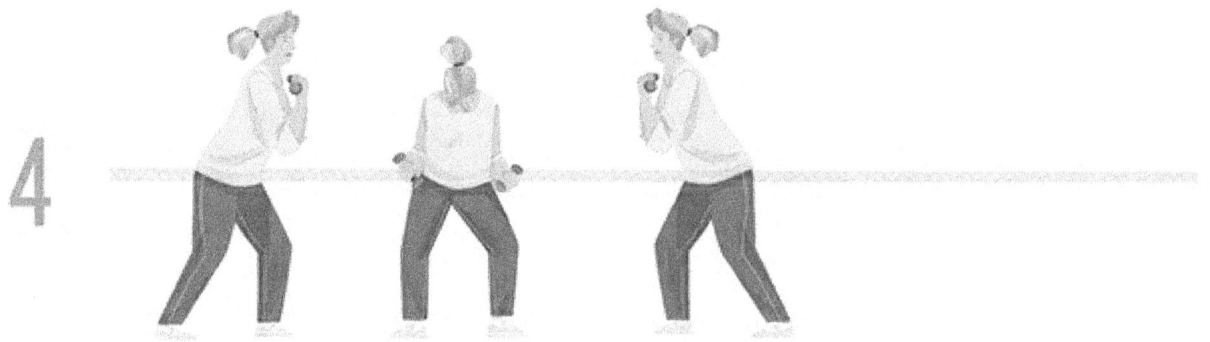

Master Gardener

ROUTINES FOR AROUND THE HOUSE

Even if you don't have a green thumb, maintaining a home usually requires some level of outdoor upkeep. This routine zeroes in on the muscles used when doing yard work.

THE ROUTINE

1 Triangle: hold for 20 to 30 seconds on each side

2 Cross Pull-Down: 8 reps on each side

3 Weighted Pull-Down: 8 reps on each side

4 Crunching Twists: 12 reps

Remember: This routine has a lot of up-and-down motion. Take it slow and steady to keep your balance, and if you become lightheaded, pause and take a rest.

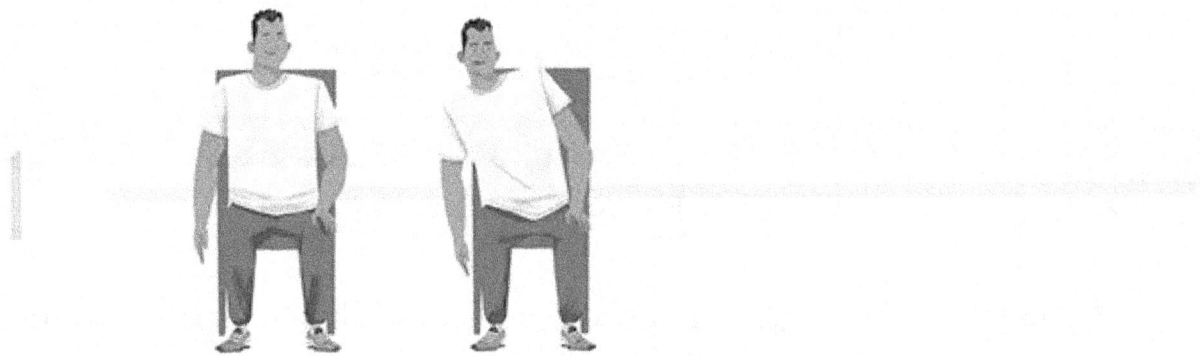

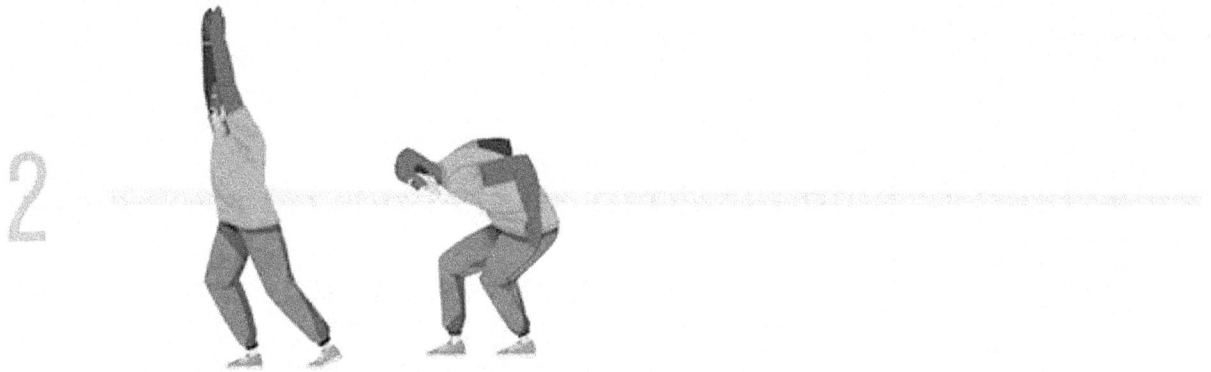

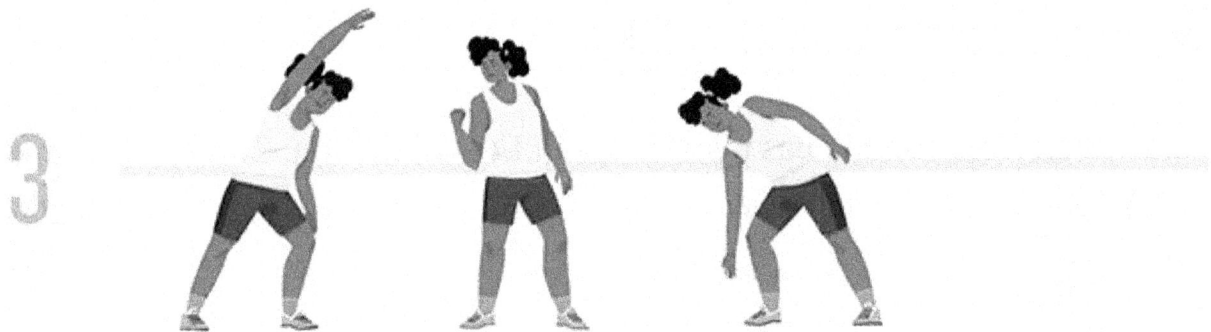

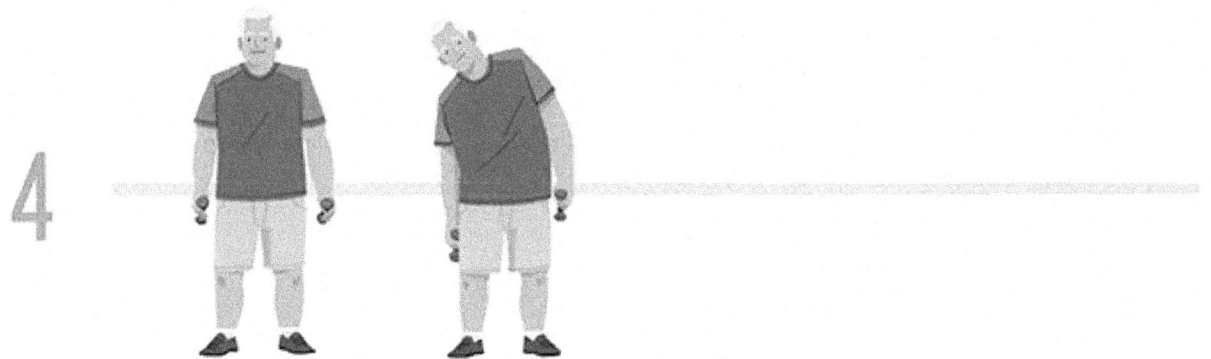

Getting Ready

ROUTINES FOR AROUND THE HOUSE

If you struggle with mobility, simply getting dressed in the morning can be very tough. This routine will help you build flexibility and stay pain-free while selecting and putting on clothes and shoes.

THE ROUTINE

1. Seated Side Bend: **8 reps on each side**
2. Diagonal Sit Back: **8 reps on each side**
3. Lunging Pull-Down: **8 reps on each side**
4. Reach Backs: **20 reps**

Remember: Moving more mindfully can help you avoid injuries. So, try to keep these moves in mind and mimic the steady, controlled motions when you're actually getting dressed. The more you build muscle memory, the more natural this will become.

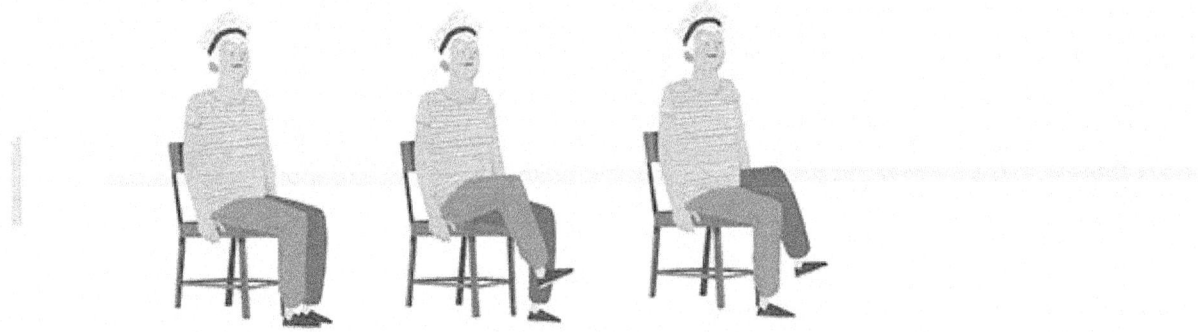

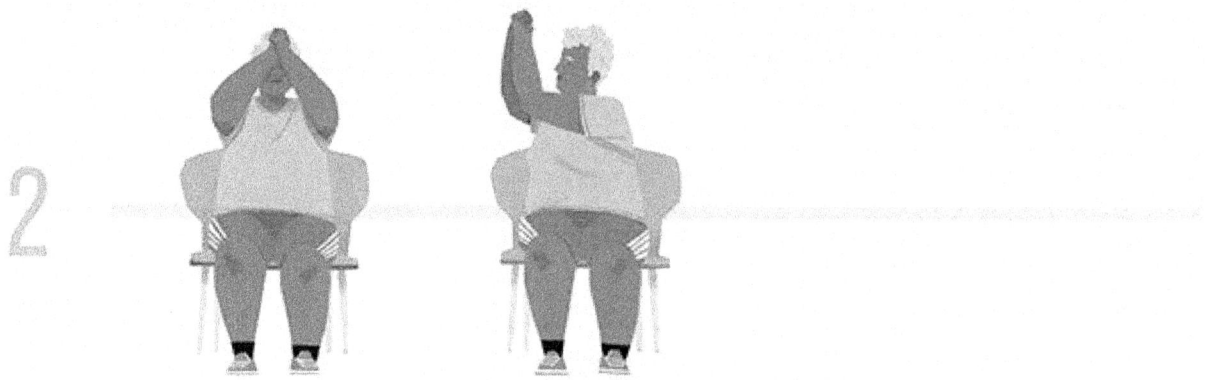

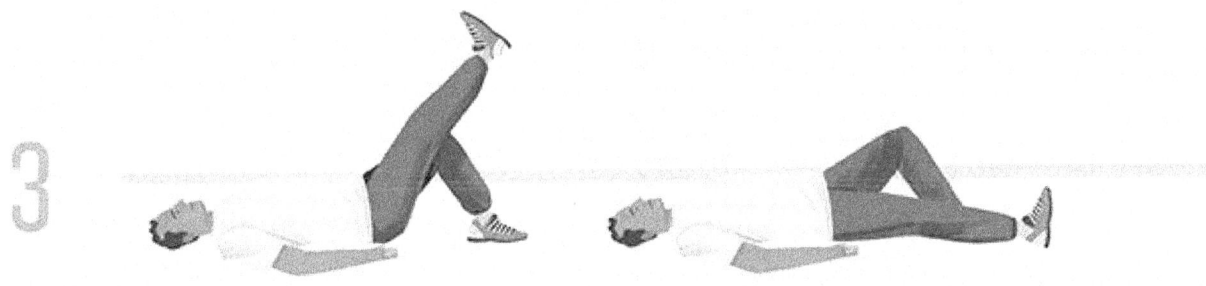

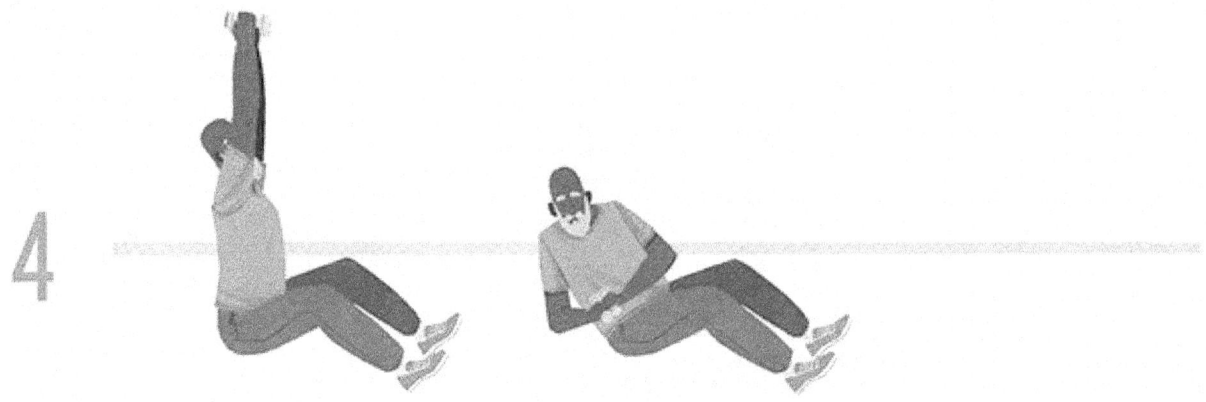

On the Move

ROUTINES FOR ACTIVE LIVING

When we talk about living a fulfilling life in your senior years, a big part of that is maintaining your independence. These exercises will help you stay mobile so you can run errands, play with your grandkids, take part in social activities, and participate in the hobbies you enjoy.

THE ROUTINE

1   Knee Lifts: **20 reps**

2   Seated Twist: **10 reps**

3   Single Leg Lifts: **8 reps on each side**

4   Angled Side Crunch: **20 reps**

Remember: Try not to hunch over during any of the exercises. Maintain a long spine and a lifted chin, keeping plenty of space (about the size of an orange) between your chin and your chest.

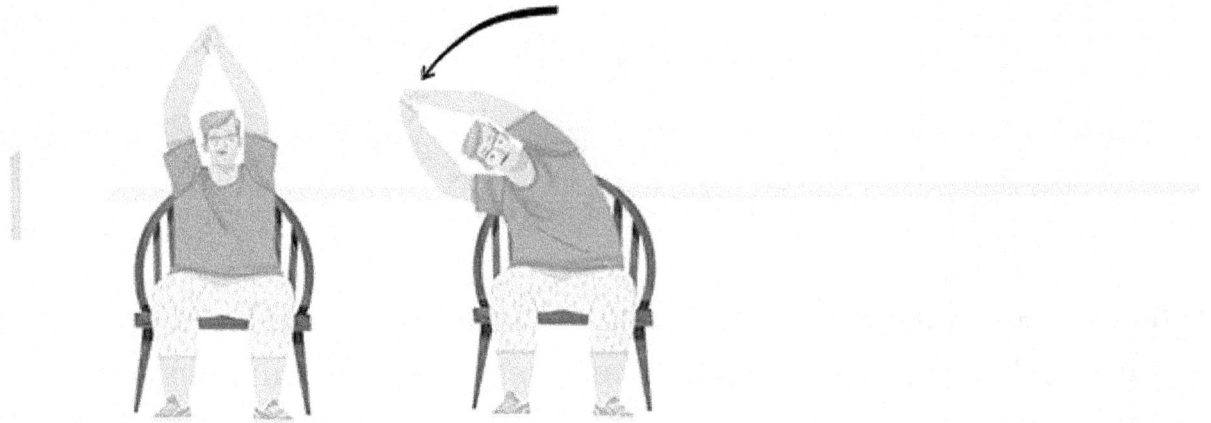

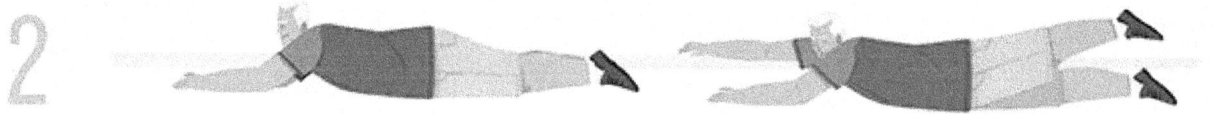

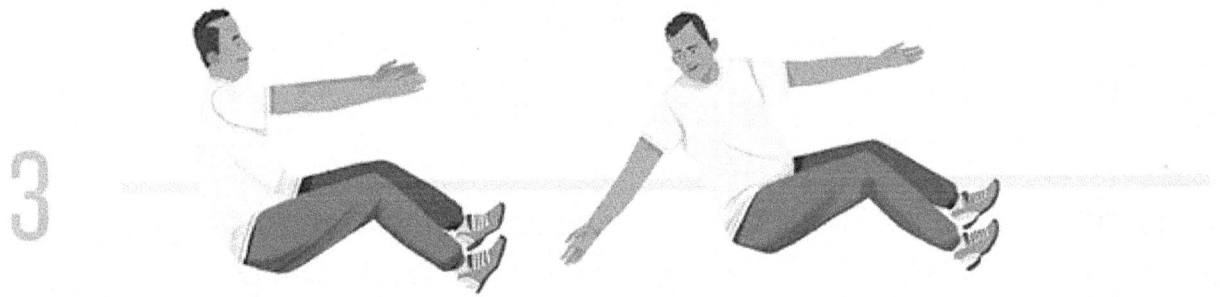

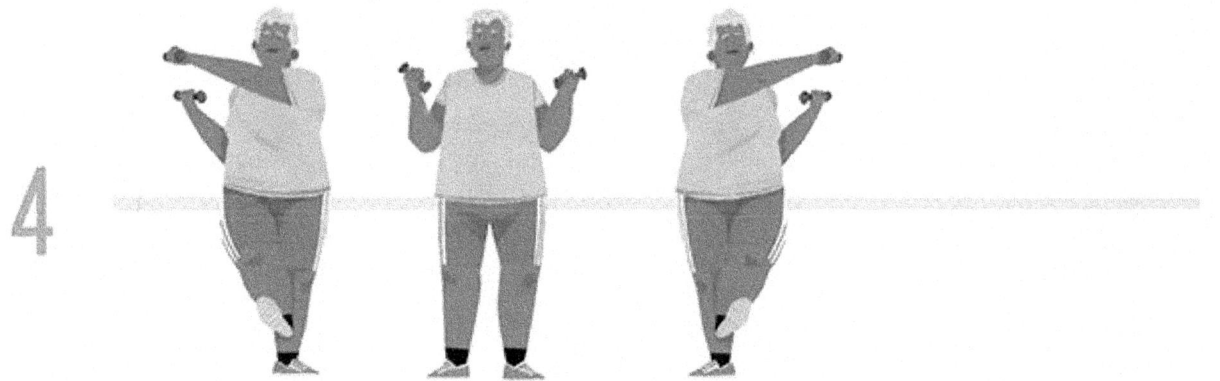

Stand Tall

ROUTINES FOR ACTIVE LIVING

It's hard to overstate the importance of proper posture in warding off pain and keeping your balance. These posture-building exercises will help you stand tall and avoid the curvature of the spine that often happens with age.

THE ROUTINE

1   Metronome: two 30-second cycles with a short break between cycles

2   Alternating Superhero: 20 reps

3   Side Sweeps: 20 reps

4   Punching Kicks: 20 reps

Remember: Your core extends beyond just the front part of your body. During the exercises, imagine drawing your midsection inward and upward from all angles, including the sides and back.

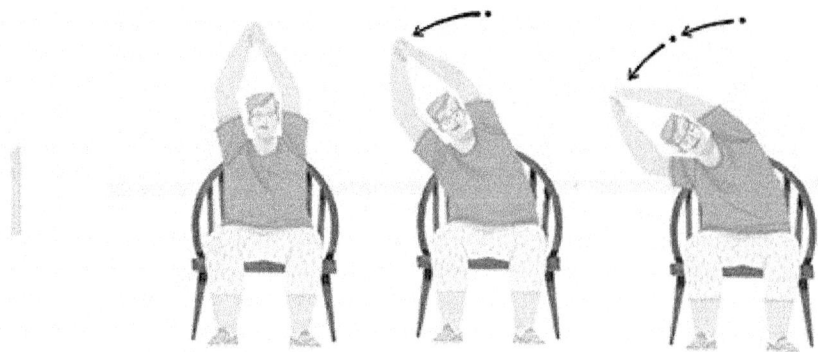

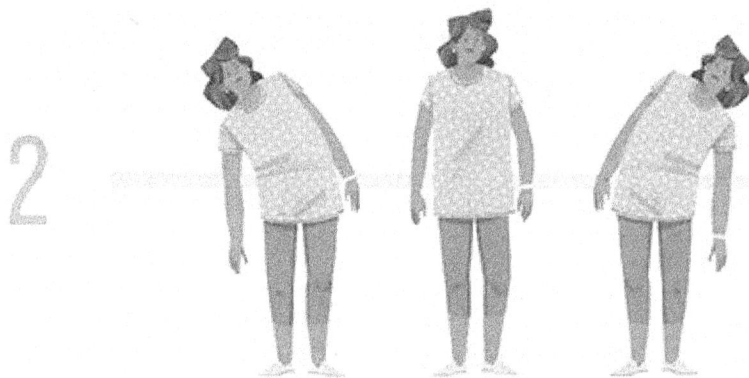

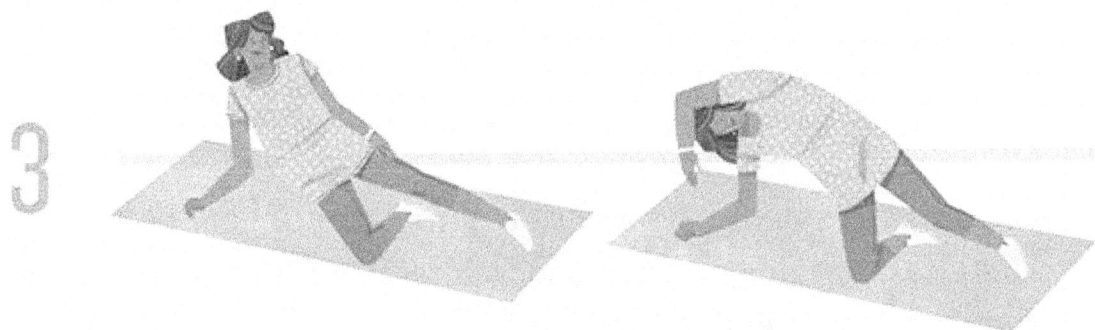

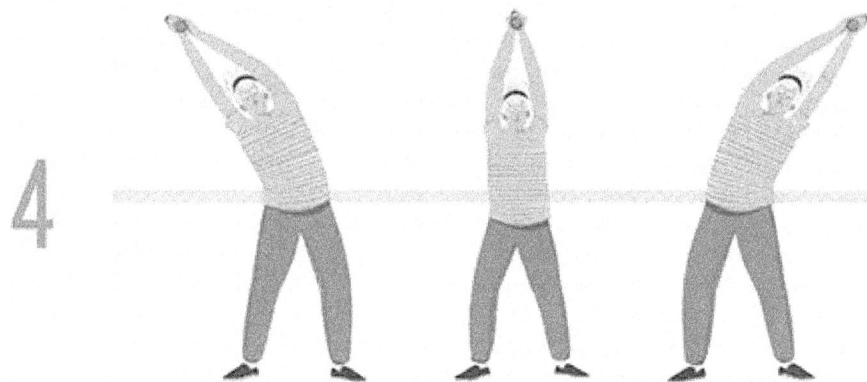

Slim and Trim

ROUTINES FOR ACTIVE LIVING

Less pain and better balance are two major benefits of a strong core, but looking and feeling your best when you're out and about is equally important. These exercises zero in on your midsection, trimming your waist and helping you feel confident in your clothes.

THE ROUTINE

1 Ticking Clock: **10 reps**

2 Side Bends: **20 reps**

3 Modified Side Plank: **hold for 20 seconds**

4 Dumbbell Side Bend: **20 reps**

Remember: You can multiply your results by making smart choices in the kitchen. Choose whole grains over refined grains, water or tea over soda and juice, and more fruits and vegetables to make even more progress in defining your waist.

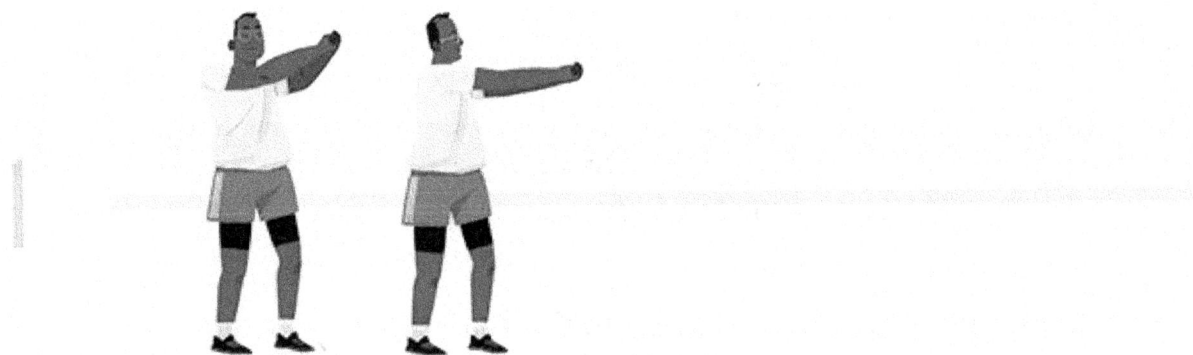

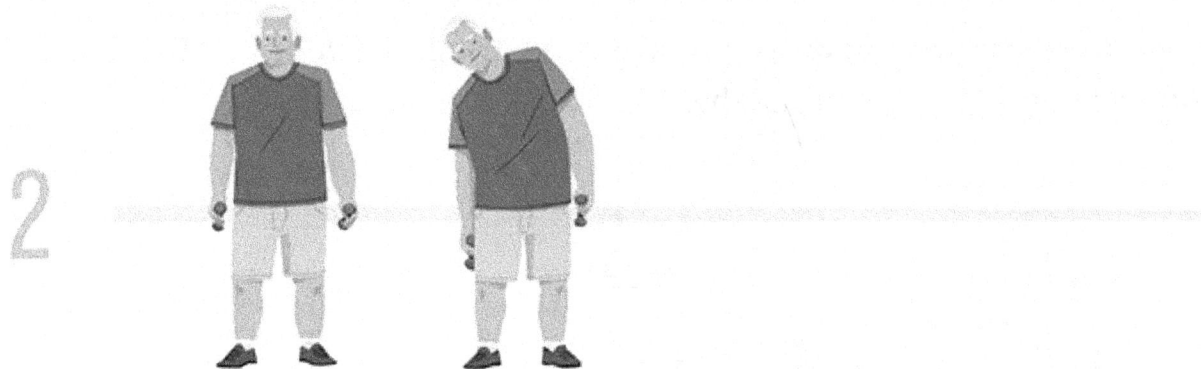

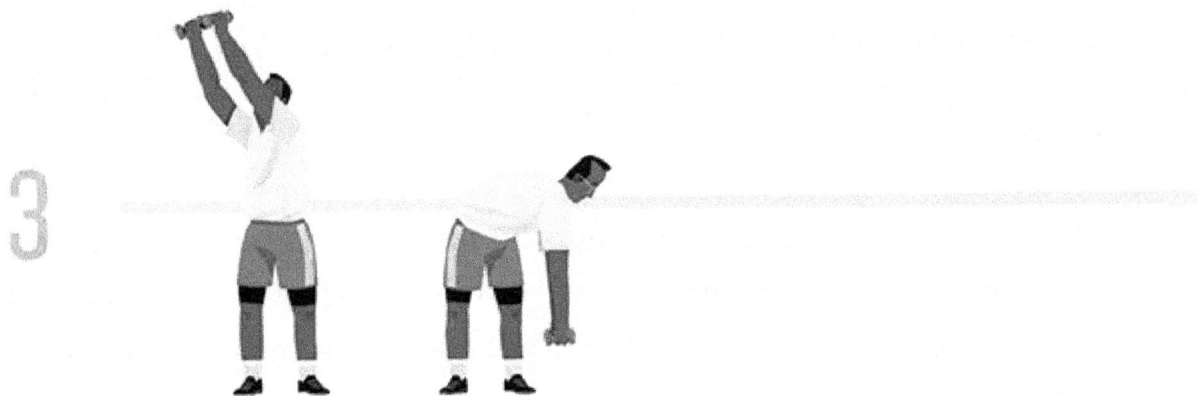

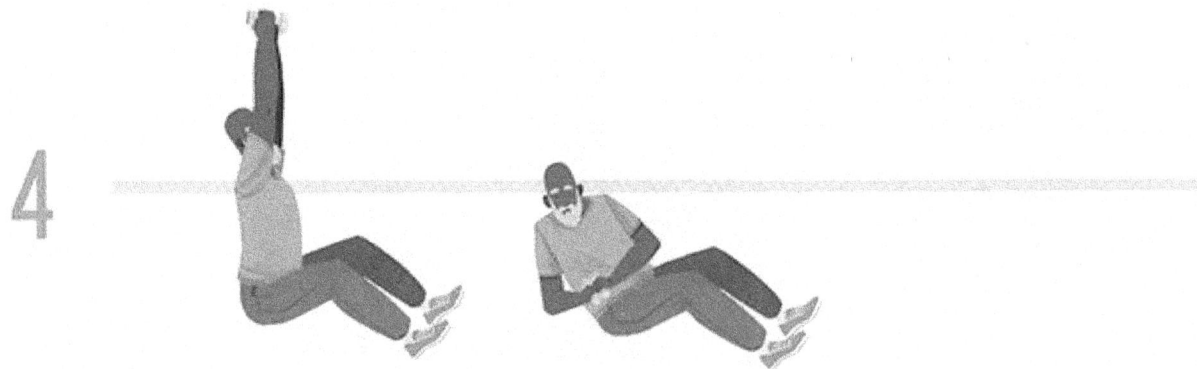

Shopping Trip

ROUTINES FOR ACTIVE LIVING

This routine is all about mastering the motions associated with a trip to the grocery store, such as picking items off the shelf, packing and unloading the car, and putting away groceries.

THE ROUTINE

1   Torso Twists: **20 reps**

2   Reach Backs: **20 reps**

3   Weighted Pull-Downs: **10 reps**

4   Angled Side Crunch: **10 reps**

Remember: Some of these exercises call for dumbbells, but you can easily substitute a medicine ball, kettlebell, or even a water bottle instead. Start with a light weight (e.g., 2 to 3 pounds) and increase the weight only if and when you feel comfortable.

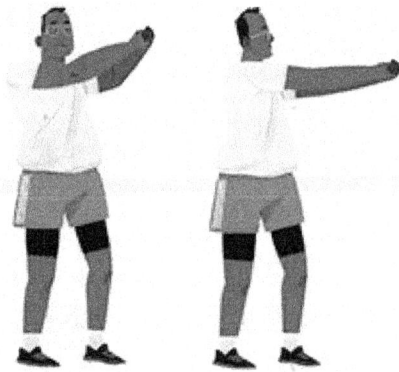

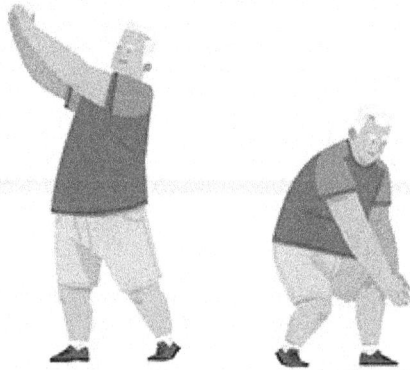

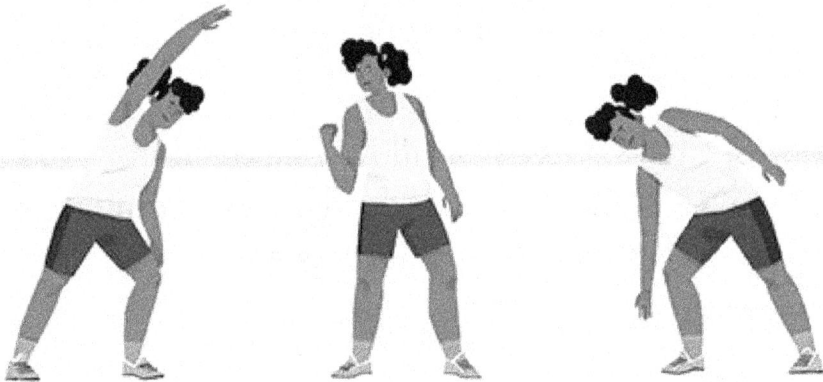

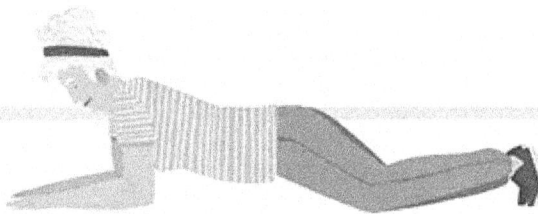

Sports Fan

ROUTINES FOR ACTIVE LIVING

Tennis, golf, racquetball, pickleball, cycling, and swimming are all excellent forms of exercise. This routine strengthens the muscles used in many of these sports and might even help you improve your game, too.

THE ROUTINE

1   Torso Twists: **20 reps**

2   Wood Chop: **10 reps on each side**

3   Lunging Pull-Down: **10 reps on each side**

4   Kneeling Plank: **hold for 20 seconds**

Remember: Don't forget to breathe. Just as when you're doing a sport, it's important to be mindful that you're taking deep, even breaths. Working on your breathing will also improve your endurance.

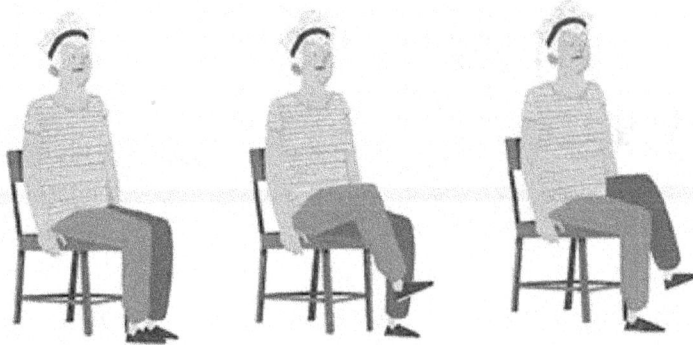

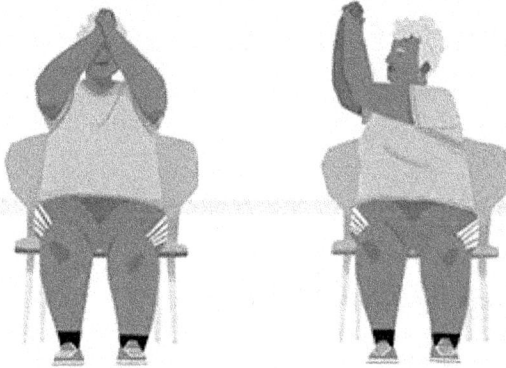

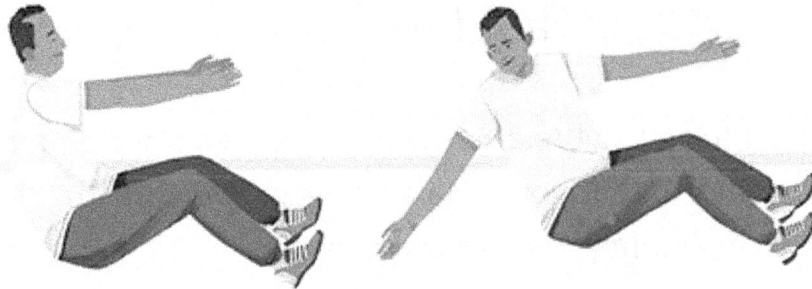

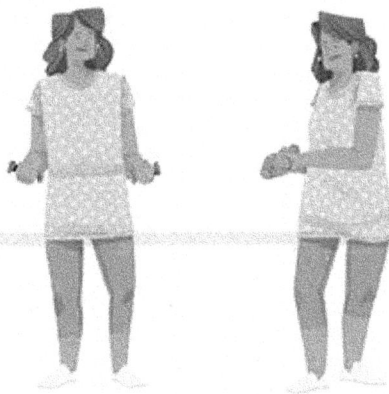

Behind the Wheel

ROUTINES FOR ACTIVE LIVING

Driving uses your core muscles more than you might think. You need a strong core to maintain a clear view of the road, pivot and check your blind spots, and get out of your vehicle safely.

THE ROUTINE

1. **Knee Lifts:** 20 reps
2. **Seated Twist:** 10 reps
3. **Side Sweeps:** 20 reps
4. **Twisting Lunge:** 8 reps on each side

Remember: Many falls happen when getting out of the car. Combine this routine with the Up and at 'Em routine, which will help you comfortably leave your vehicle.

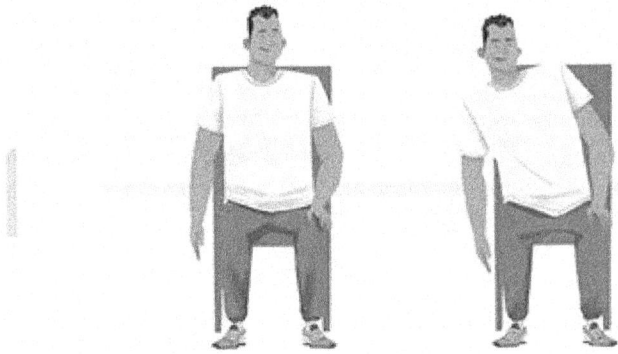

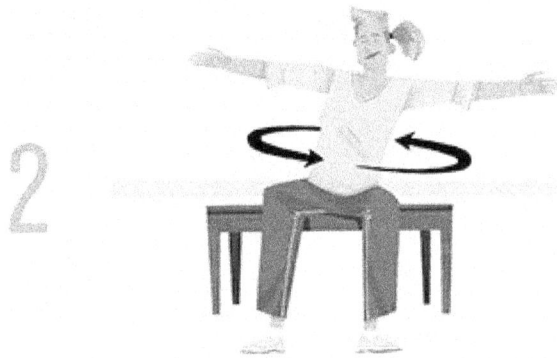

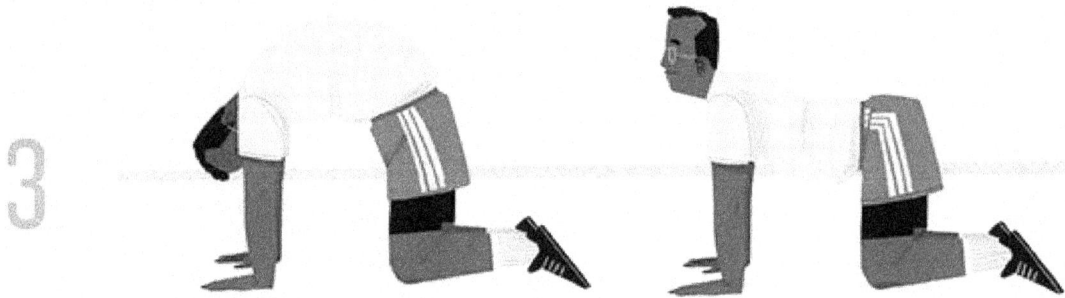

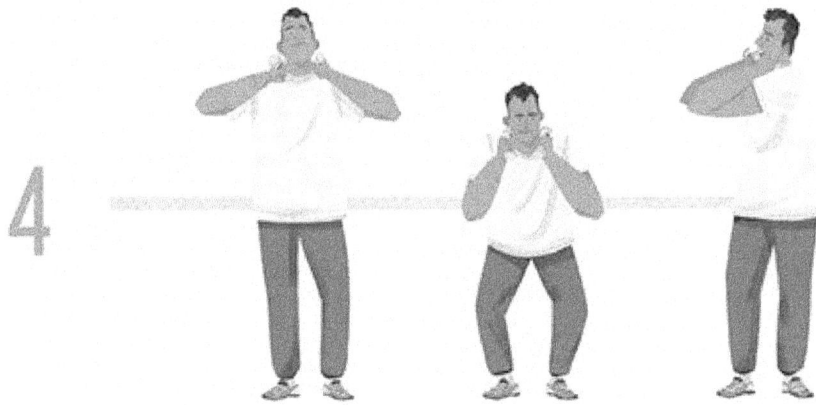

Lower Back Pain

ROUTINES FOR ACHES AND PAINS

As we've discussed throughout this book, lower back pain is often the result of a weak core, which throws your spine out of alignment. This routine will build core strength and improve your posture while relieving the tension on the muscles surrounding your spine.

THE ROUTINE

1   Seated Side Bend: **8 reps on each side**

2   Ab Circles: **10 circles on each side**

3   Cat Cow: **10 cycles**

4   Squat with Twist: **20 reps**

Remember: The Ab Circles and Cat Cow moves should feel great in addition to building strength. Take your time and breathe deeply while making these moves. If you feel comfortable doing more than the suggested number of reps, go for it!

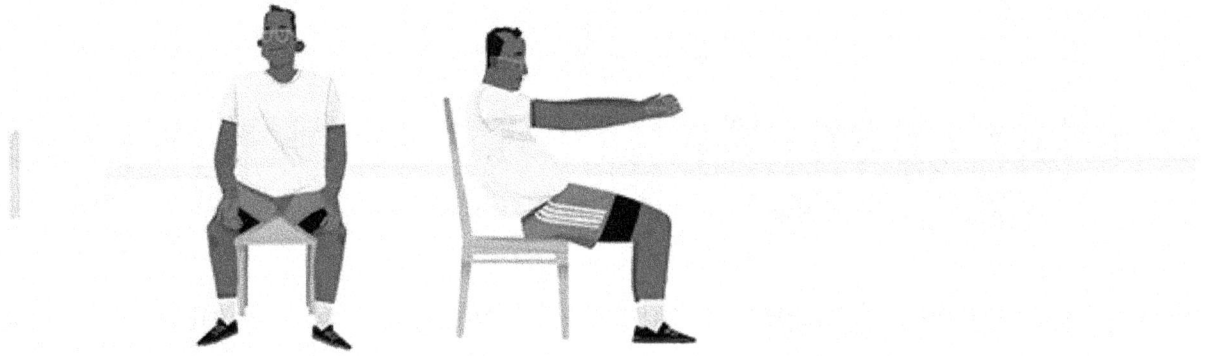

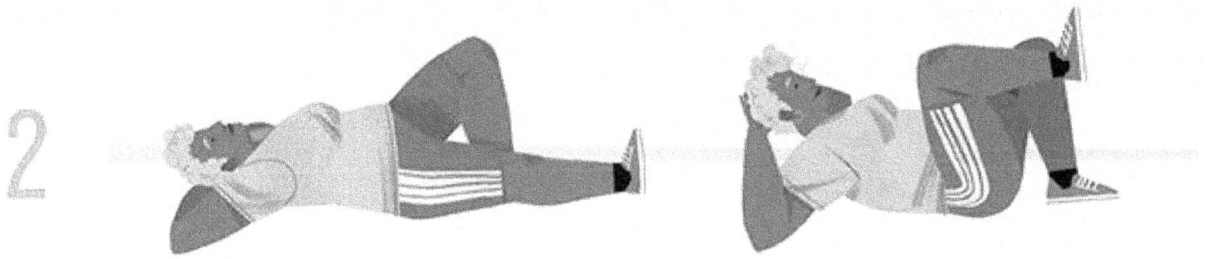

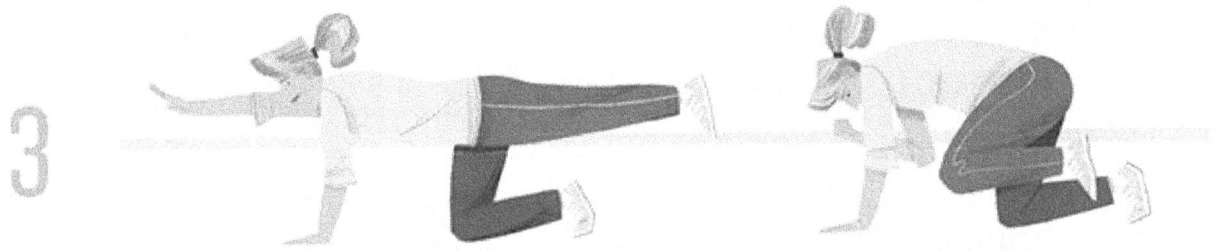

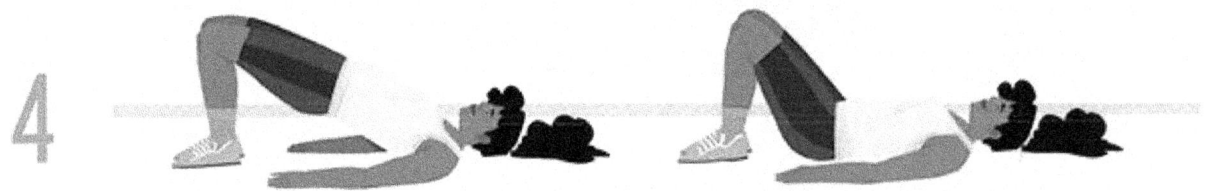

Lower Back Pain II

ROUTINES FOR ACHES AND PAINS

This routine works your hip muscles in addition to strengthening the abdominal wall. It's all connected; looser, stronger hips will also help reduce tension in your lower back.

THE ROUTINE

1 Slow Recline: **10 reps**

2 One-Legged Crunch: **8 reps on each side**

3 Bird Dog: **8 reps on each side**

4 Bridge: **10 reps**

Remember: Though it may feel counterintuitive, try not to squeeze your glutes while doing the Bridge move. The work of lifting your midsection should be done by your core and hips. Pressing your feet into the floor will help with this.

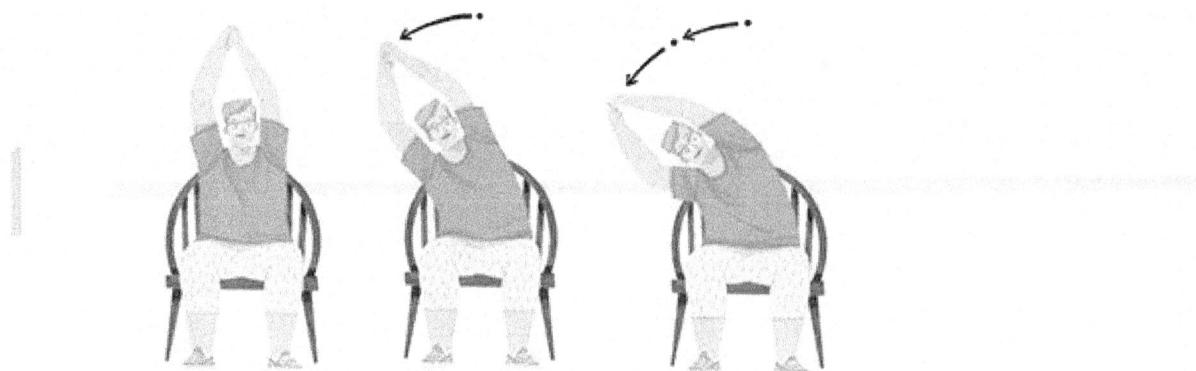

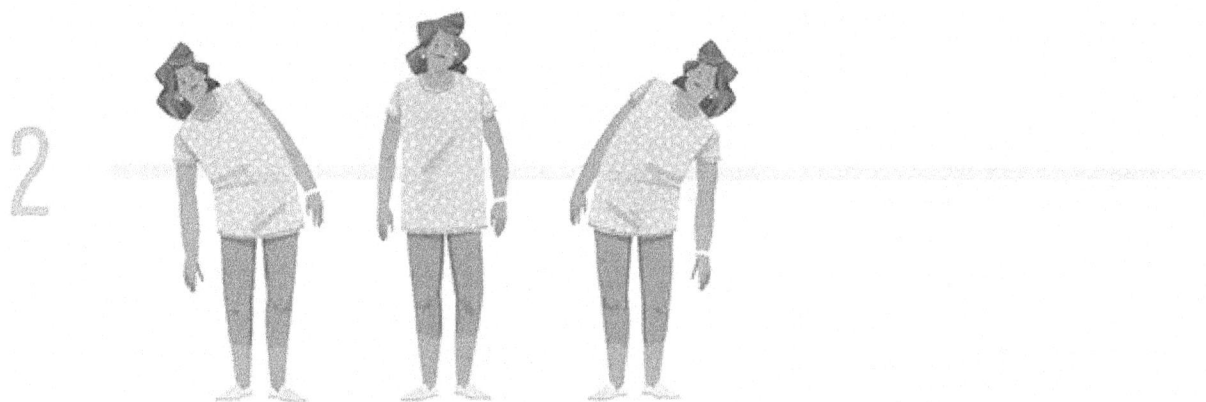

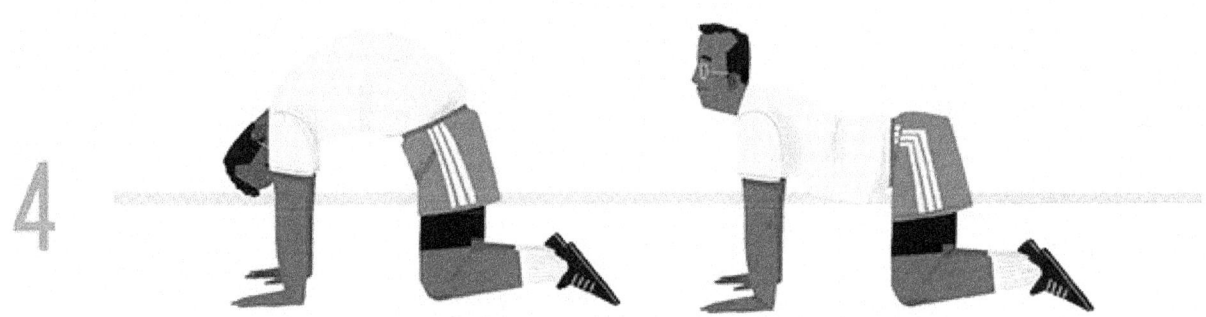

Achy Spine

ROUTINES FOR ACHES AND PAINS

The muscles that run along your spine are so important for keeping you in proper alignment and, in turn, pain free. This routine strengthens and lengthens those muscles, which will help you avoid the "hunched" look in addition to relieving spine pain.

THE ROUTINE

1 Ticking Clock: **10 reps**

2 Side Bends: **20 reps**

3 Alternating Superhero: **20 reps**

4 Cat Cow: **10 cycles**

Remember: To avoid straining your neck, avoid the urge to look forward while doing the Alternating Superhero move. Instead, keep your gaze straight down toward the floor with a neutral spine.

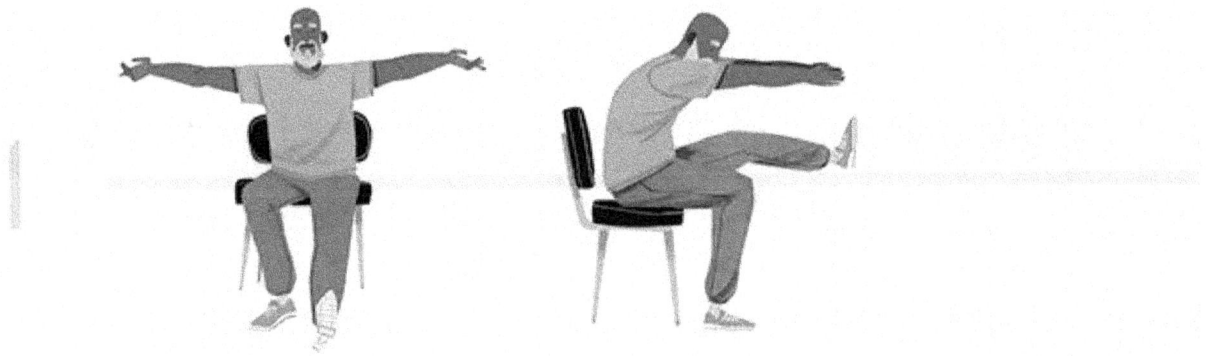

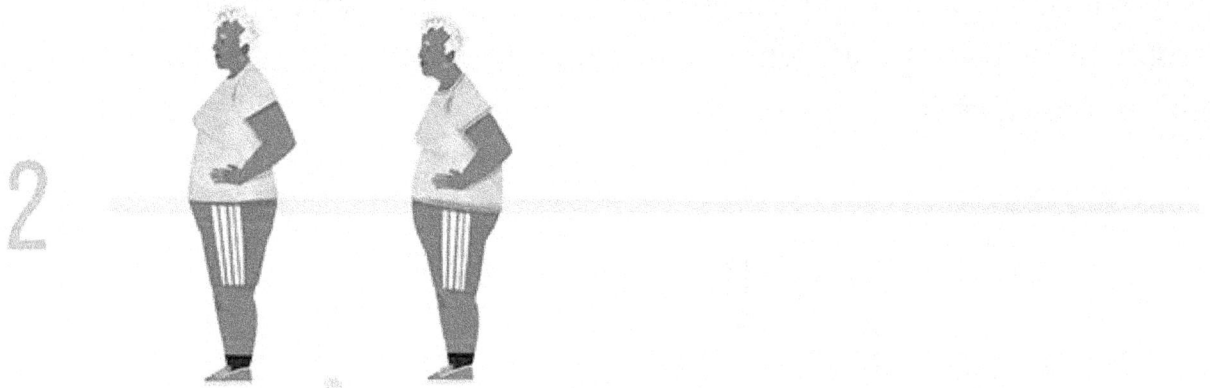

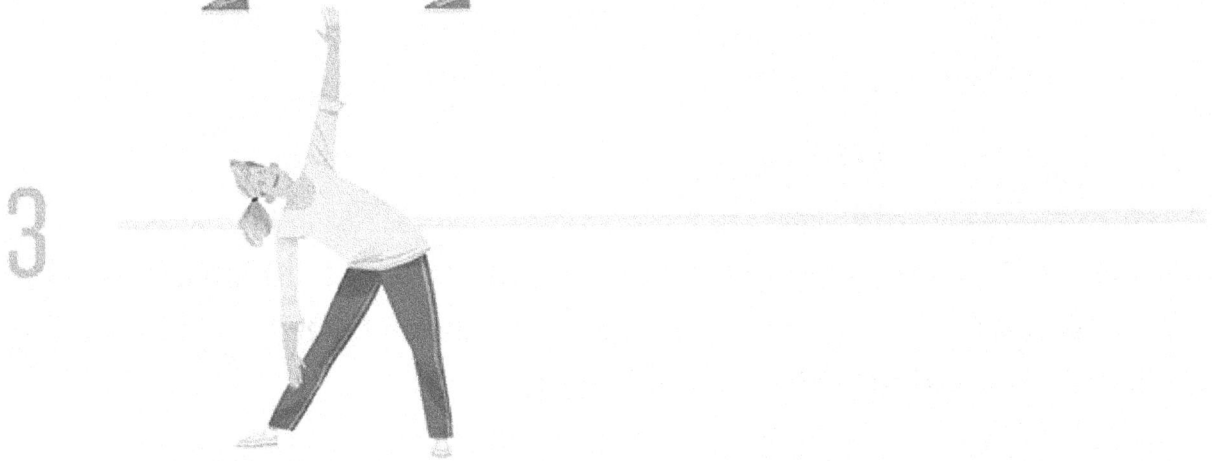

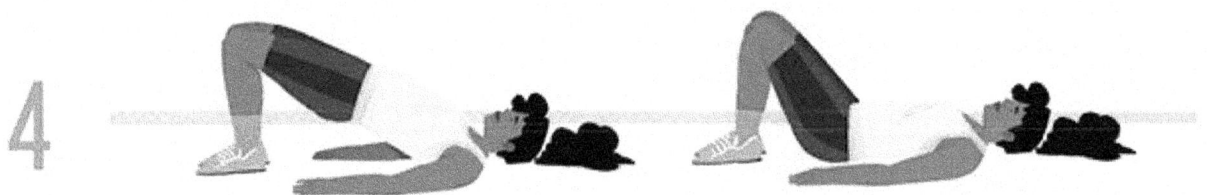

Hip Pain

ROUTINES FOR ACHES AND PAINS

Many people spend eight hours a day or more sitting down, which can really do a number on your hips. This routine brings movement and blood flow to the area to keep your hip joints lubricated and strong.

THE ROUTINE

1   Straight Leg Crunch: **8 reps on each side**

2   Pelvic Tilt: **15 reps**

3   Triangle: **hold for 20 to 30 seconds on each side**

4   Bridge: **10 reps**

Remember: If you work at a desk, this is a great routine to use in the middle of the day to give your hips a break. Try pairing this routine with a short walk for some welcome midday pain relief.

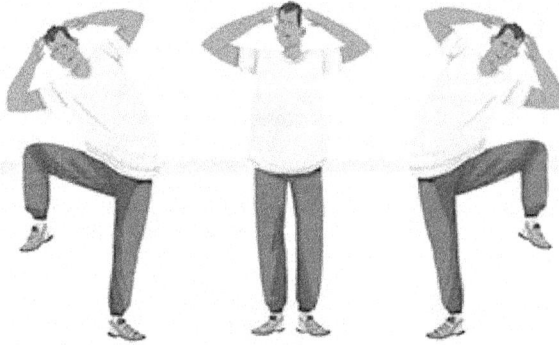

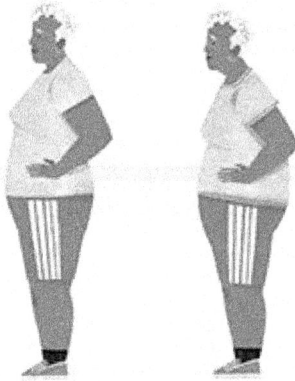

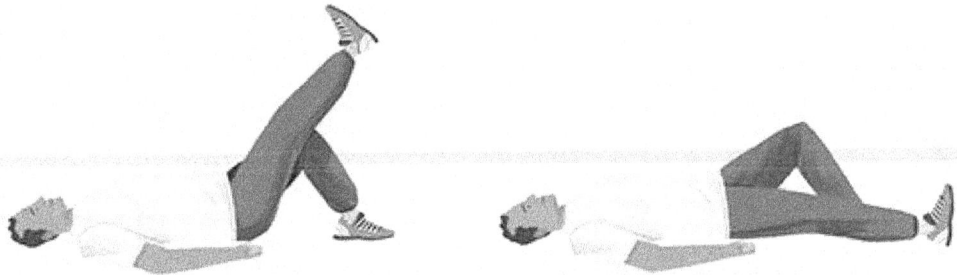

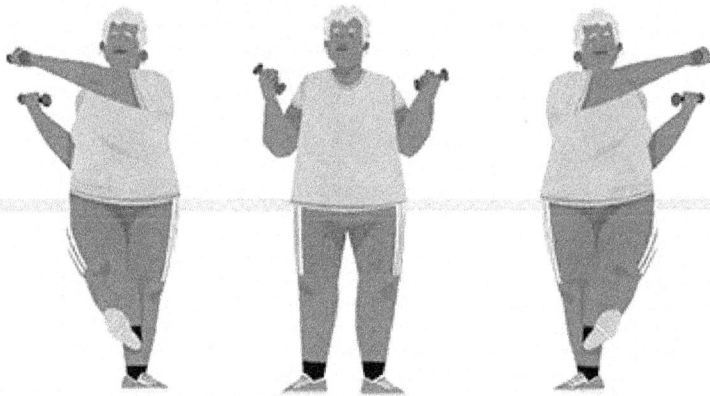

Strong Hip Flexors

ROUTINES FOR ACHES AND PAINS

Along with the other core muscles, the hip flexors stabilize the pelvis and spine and help you move with a lower risk of injury. If you feel pain or a pulling sensation when lifting your leg toward your chest, as when walking up stairs, it's a sign you might want to work on strengthening your hip flexors.

THE ROUTINE

1 Side Crunch with Leg Lift: **8 reps on each side**

2 Pelvic Tilt: **15 reps**

3 Single Leg Lifts: **8 reps on each side**

4 Punching Kicks: **20 reps**

Remember: If you're not used to working your hip flexors, these exercises may be quite uncomfortable at first. A little discomfort is normal, but stop if you feel pain.

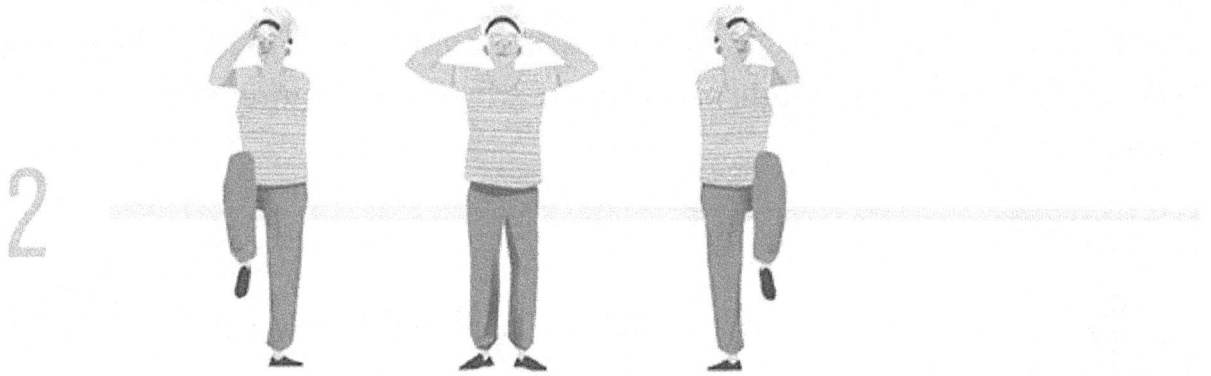

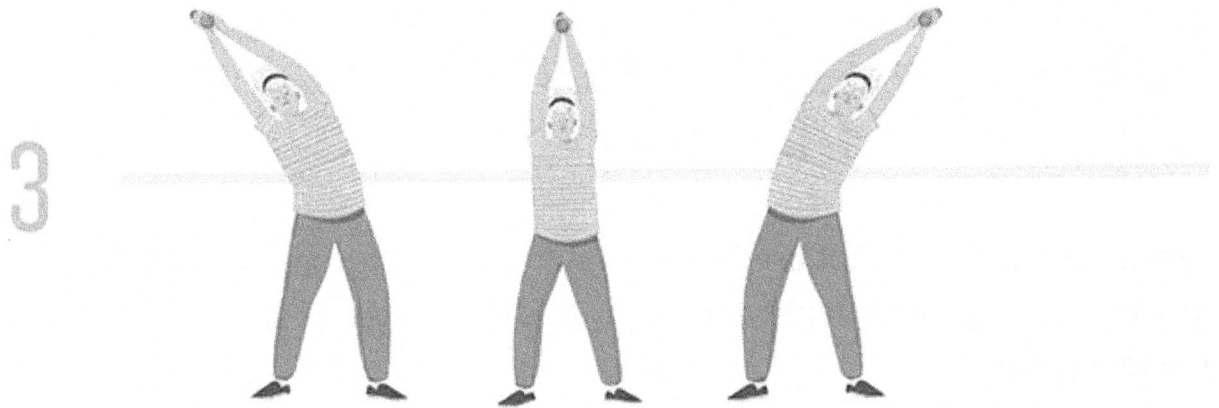

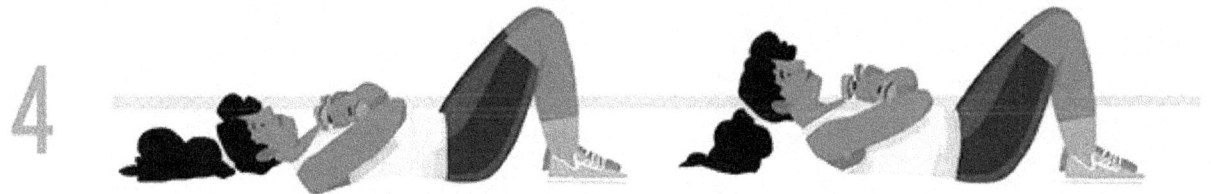

Strong Joints

ROUTINES FOR ACHES AND PAINS

Experiencing a dull ache in your hips or knees? Then you're no stranger to joint pain. If left unattended, joint pain can range from annoying to downright debilitating. The weights incorporated into this routine will help you maintain strong bones and pain-free joints.

THE ROUTINE

1   Ab Circles: 10 circles on each side

2   Standing Crunch: 20 reps

3   Dumbbell Side Bend: 20 reps

4   Weighted Crunch: 20 reps

Remember: Start with a low amount of weight (e.g., two to three pounds) and increase the weight only if you feel comfortable. Working consistently with light weights is fine, too!

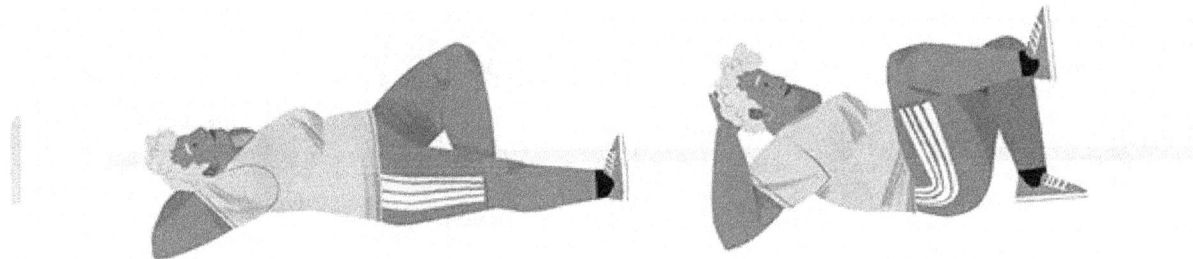

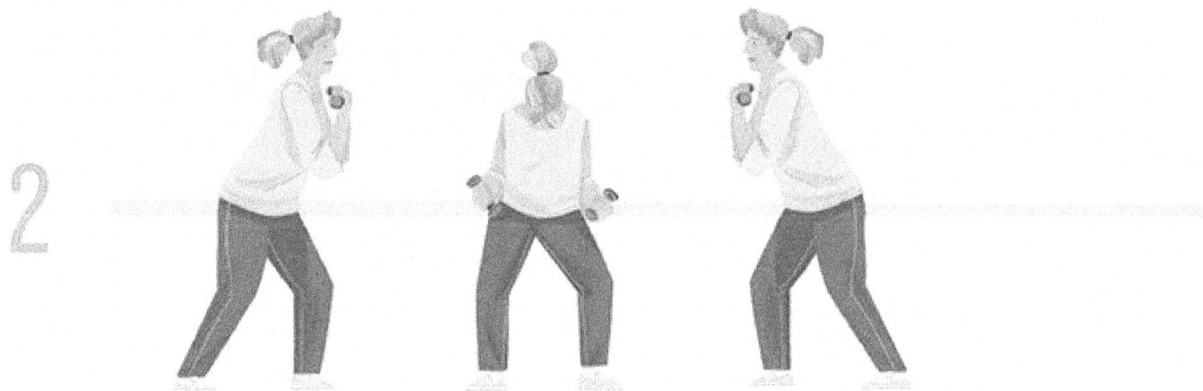

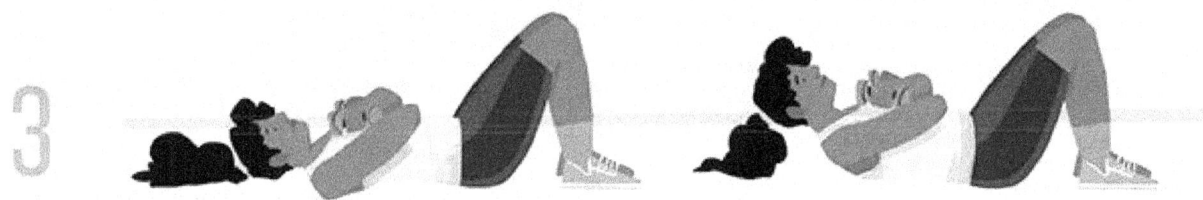

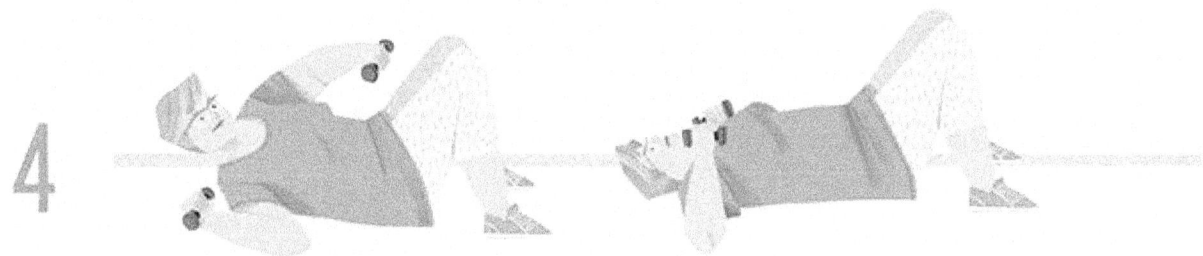

Calorie Burn

ROUTINES TO DO WITH A PARTNER

One of the best ways to get a bigger calorie burn from your workout is by adding weights and using your own body weight to increase the resistance. This routine will challenge your muscles and get your heart rate up, which contributes to burning fat. To test whether you're working in the target intensity range, try doing this routine with a friend while keeping up a conversation. You may feel a bit out of breath, but you should be able to keep chatting. If you feel so winded it's tough to speak, stop and take a breather.

THE ROUTINE

1 One-Legged Crunch: 10 reps on each side

2 Crunching Twists: 12 reps

3 Weighted Crunch: 20 reps

4 Punching Crunch: 20 reps

Remember: If this is too challenging, ease your way into it by doing the exercises without weights at first. You can also try using soup cans, which are light and easy to hold.

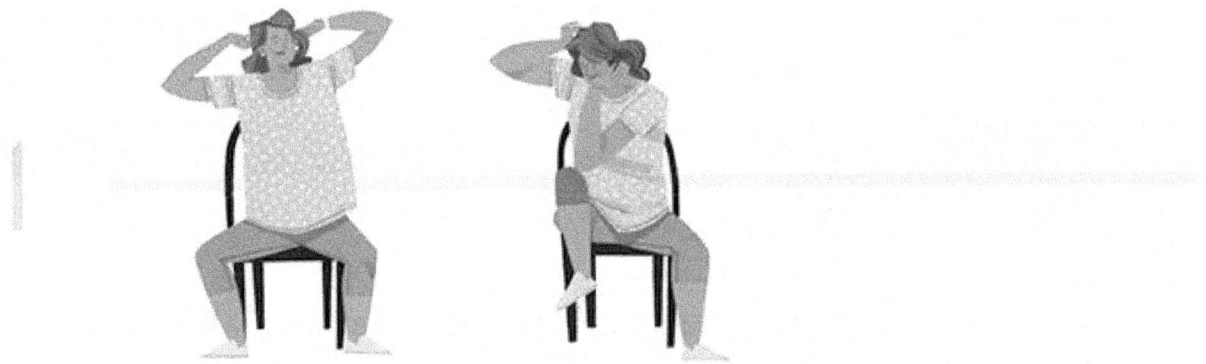

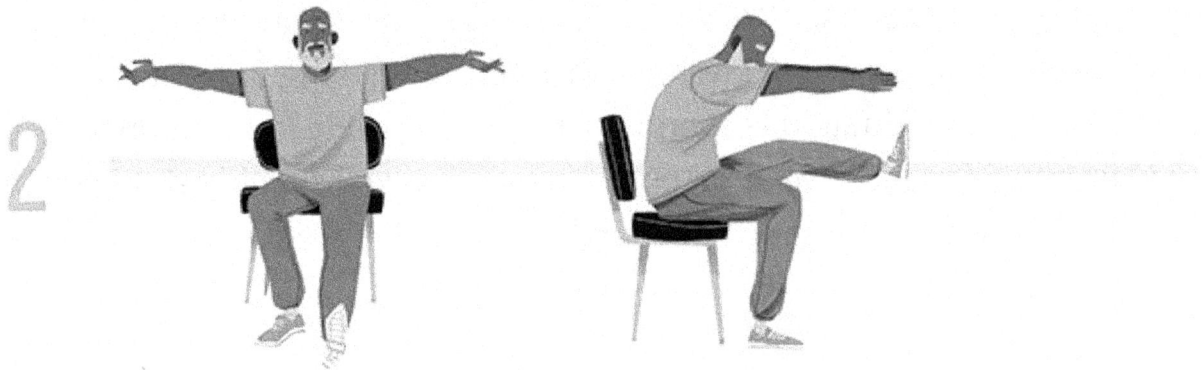

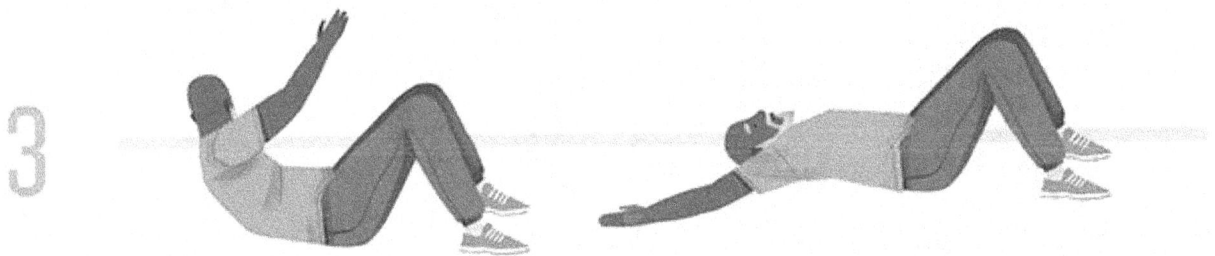

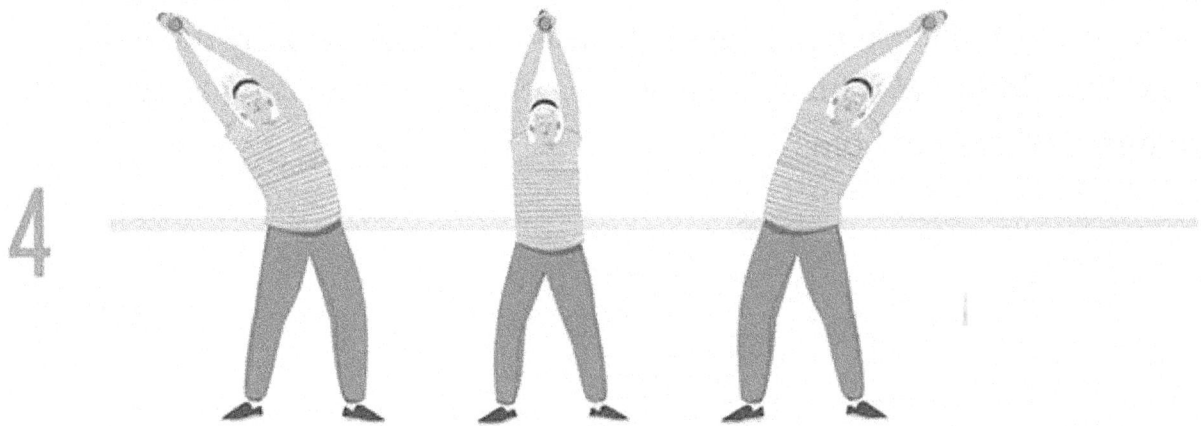

Core Blaster

ROUTINES TO DO WITH A PARTNER

We've talked a lot about how the core wraps around your entire midsection, but we know you likely really want to focus on flattening your stomach. This routine zeroes in on the rectus abdominis and transverse abdominis muscles to help you do just that. Having a workout buddy is a surefire way to hold yourself accountable and push yourself to new accomplishments. Try this routine with a friend and challenge each other to add a few additional reps every time you meet.

THE ROUTINE

1 Diagonal Crunch: **20 reps**

2 Straight Leg Crunch: **10 reps on each side**

3 Lever Crunch: **10 reps on each side**

4 Dumbbell Side Bend: **15 reps**

Remember: You may be crunching, but you need to be mindful that you're not crunching your neck. Keep your chin up and your neck long. Your head only needs to come a few inches off the floor, unlike when doing a full sit-up.

1

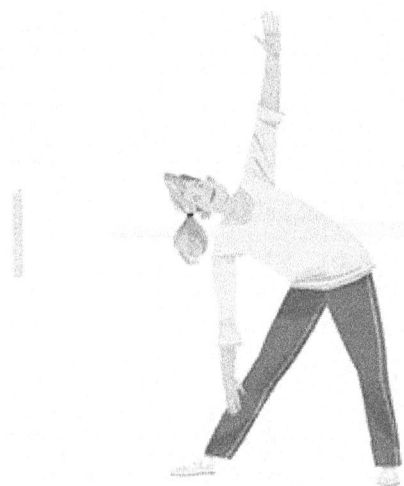

2

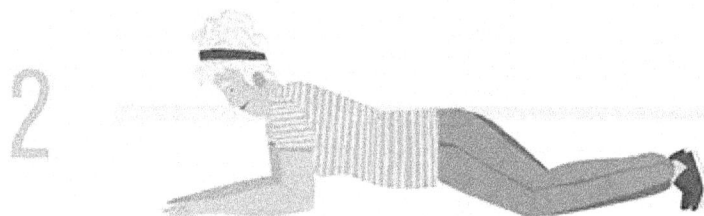

3

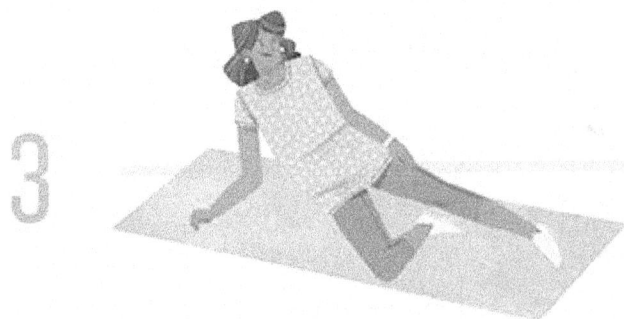 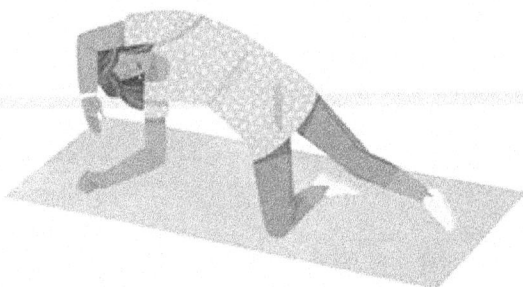

4

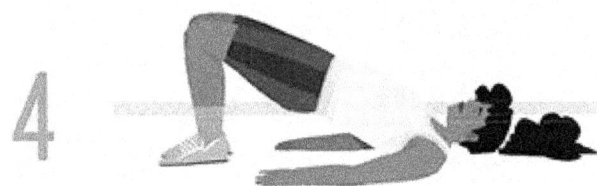 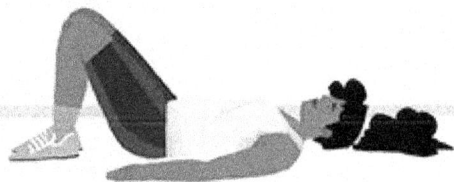

Endurance Builder

ROUTINES TO DO WITH A PARTNER

Static exercises, which are those where you're holding a position rather than repeating a move, are some of the best to help you build strength while avoiding injuries. This routine will test your stamina while helping you feel the burn. Since proper positioning is especially important with these moves, this is an ideal routine to do with a partner so you can keep an eye on each other's form.

THE ROUTINE

1   **Triangle**: hold for 30 seconds on each side

2   **Kneeling Plank**: hold for 30 seconds, take a short break, then hold for 30 seconds more

3   **Modified Side Plank**: hold for 30 seconds, take a short break, then hold for 30 seconds more

4   **Bridge**: 10 reps, holding each rep for 3 to 4 seconds at the top

Remember: Challenge yourself, building up the duration of the exercise each time you do the routine. With time, you may be able to work up to a minute in each plank pose. Even though you're holding the position, don't forget to keep breathing!

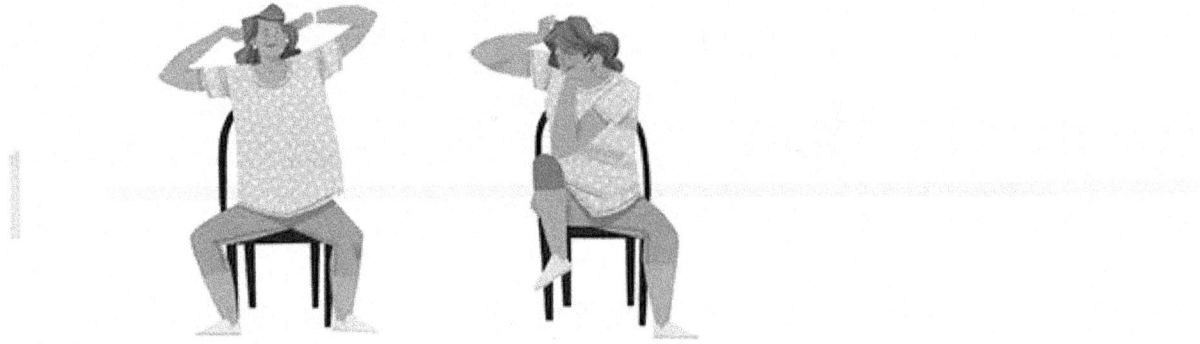

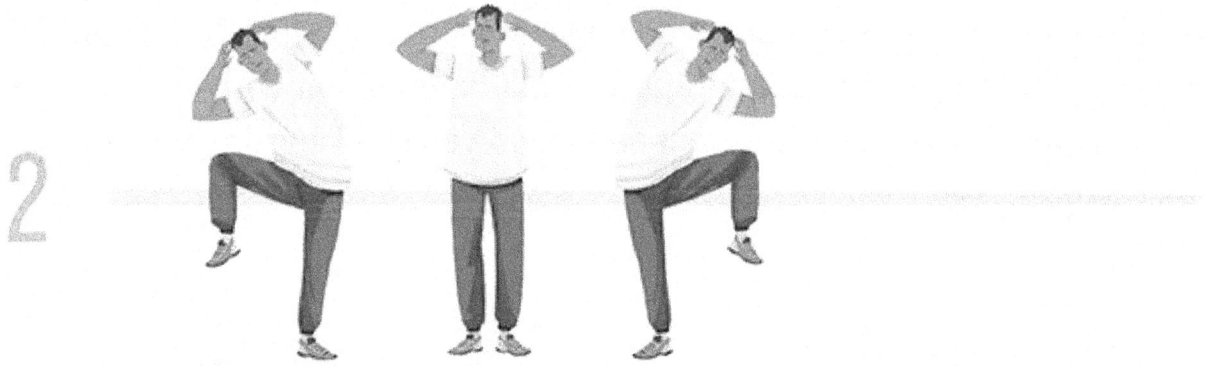

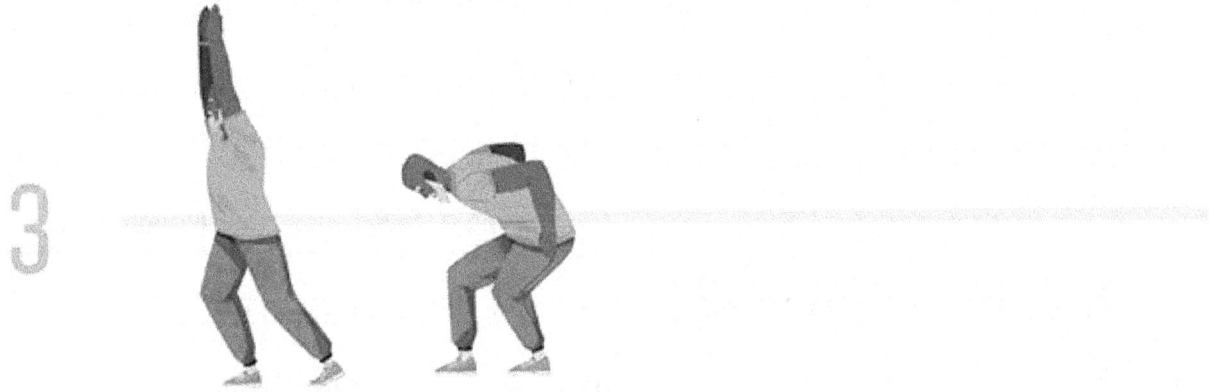

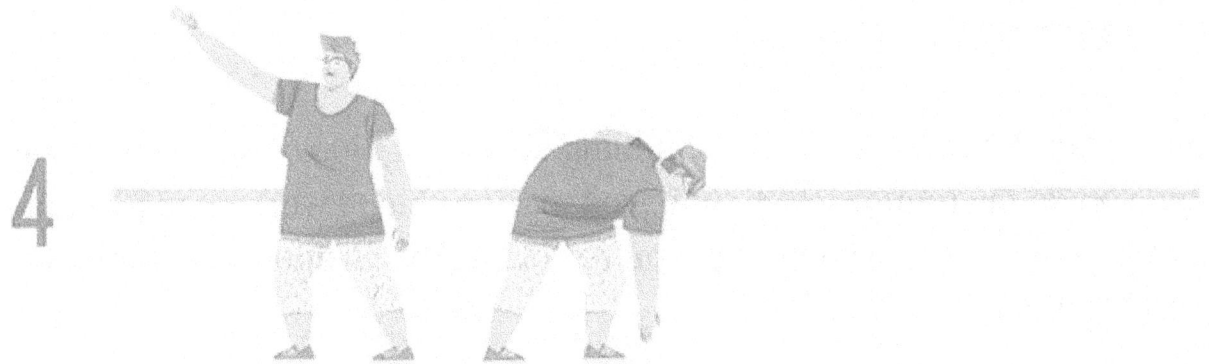

Dancing Machine

ROUTINES TO DO WITH A PARTNER

Salsa, bachata or merengue, anyone? For those of you who like to dance, this routine will help you stay light and steady on your feet through all your fancy footwork. Grab a partner who is game for trying some new moves, and work through this routine together. Exercising is a great way to get some social interaction while also doing something good for your body.

THE ROUTINE

1   Diagonal Crunch: **20 reps**

2   Side Crunch with Leg Lift: **8 reps on each side**

3   Diagonal Sit Back: **8 reps on each side**

4   Cross Pull-Down: **8 reps on each side**

Remember: With the instructions for each exercise, you'll find modifications to increase the difficulty if you're looking for more of a challenge. You can also increase the number of reps or repeat the routine in its entirety.

1

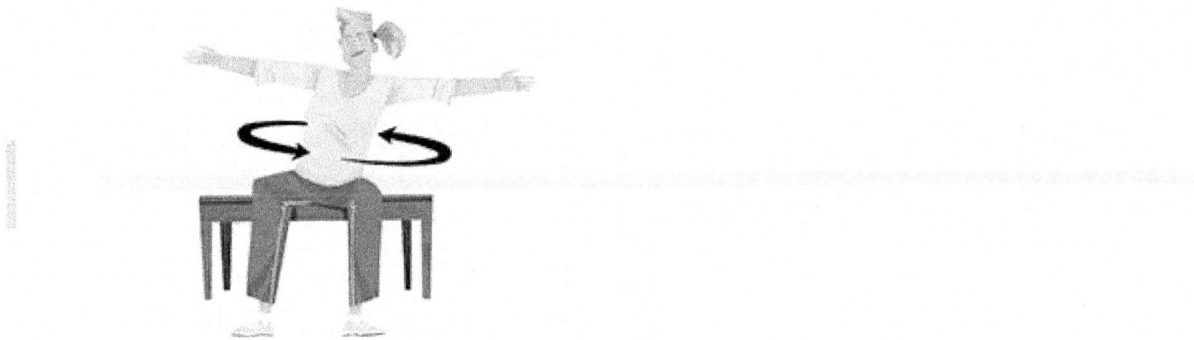

2

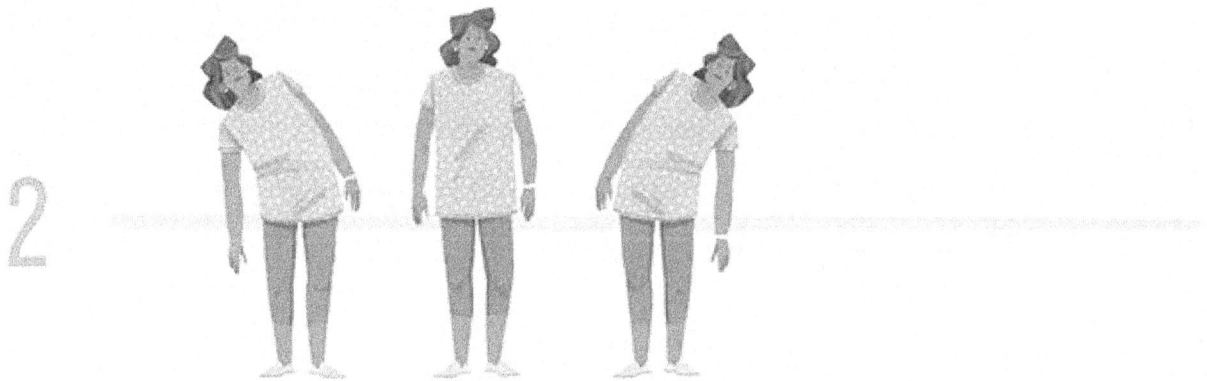

3

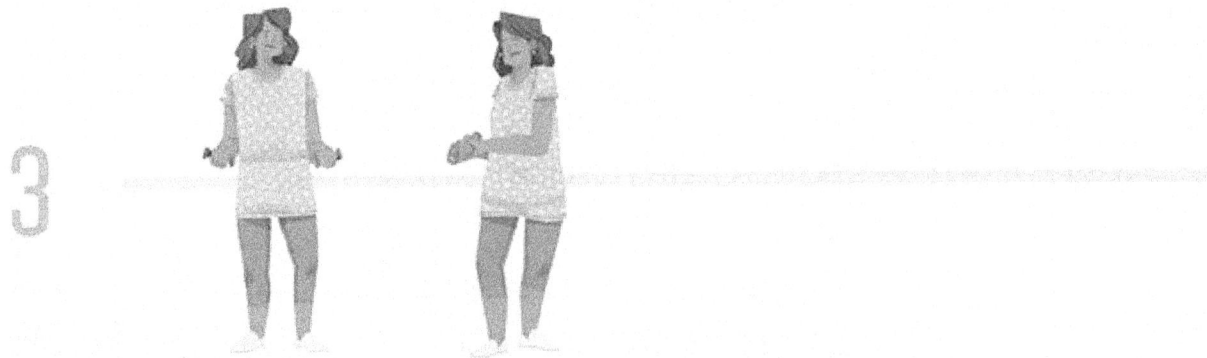

4

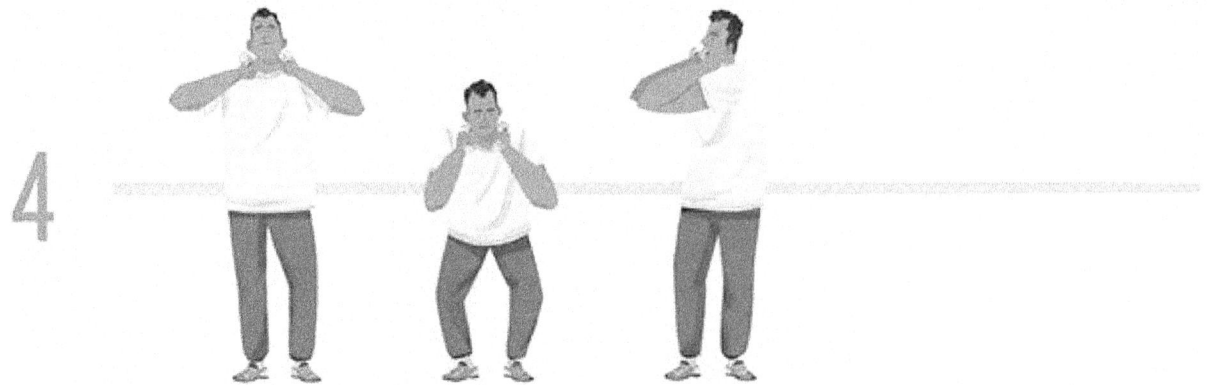

Travel Buddy

ROUTINES TO DO WITH A PARTNER

From lifting your suitcase and wheeling it through the airport to getting on and off a plane, traveling isn't easy on the body. This routine will help you maintain the strength you need to see the world comfortably. This is one of the more challenging routines in the book, so try it with a friend and encourage each other to finish strong.

THE ROUTINE

1   Ab Circles: **10 circles on each side**

2   Side Bends: **20 reps**

3   Twisting Lunge: **8 reps on each side**

4   Squat with Twist: **20 reps**

Remember: If you're a travel lover, the On the Move routine is another great set of exercises to help you stay mobile and independent.

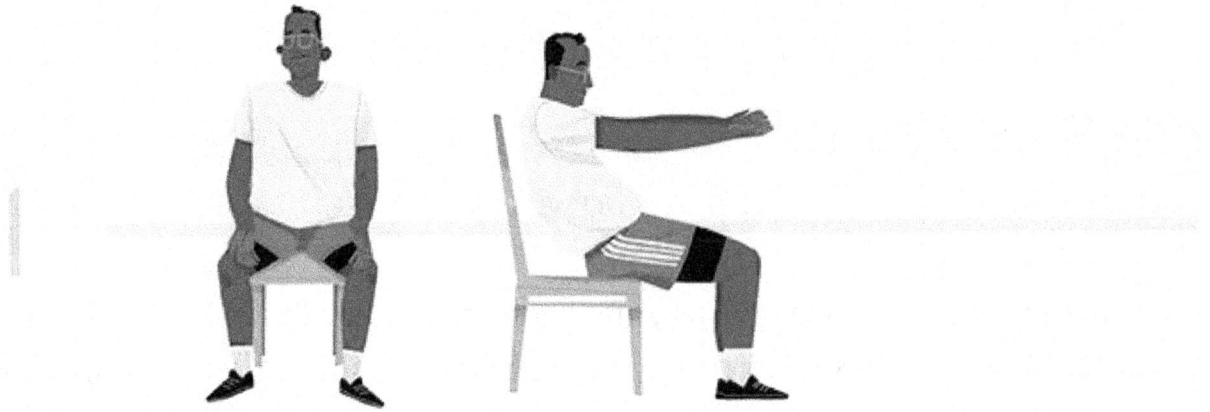

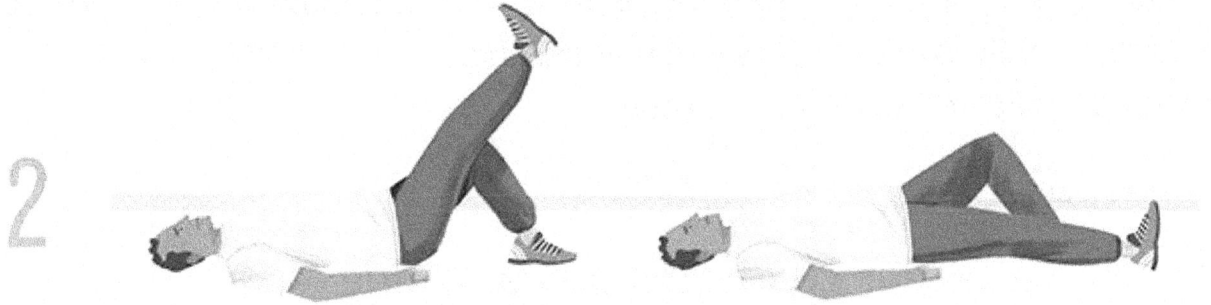

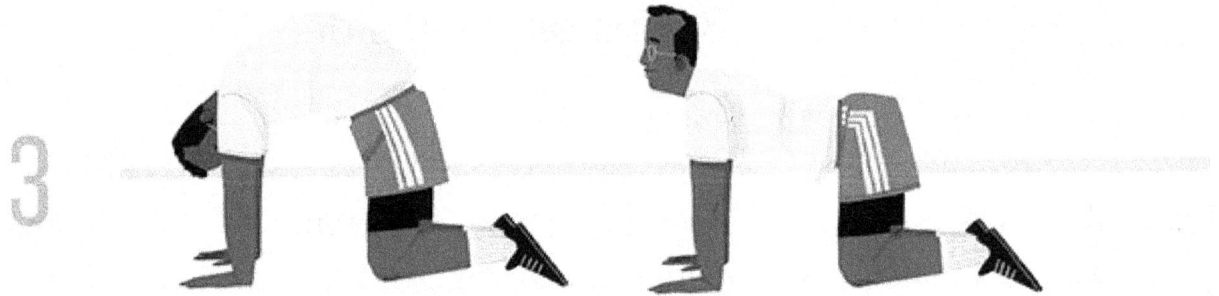

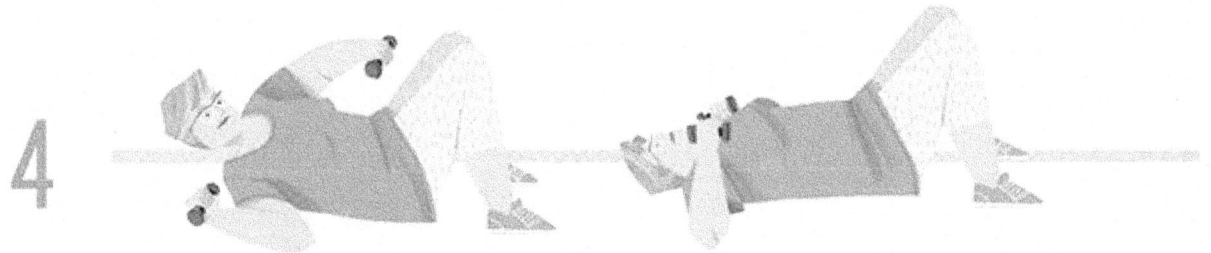

Beautiful Morning

ROUTINES TO DO WITH A PARTNER

How you feel when you wake up can have a big effect on your entire day. Start the day on a high note and use this routine to help you get out of bed pain free every day. While you're at it, why not ask your spouse or a family member to join you and enjoy a few moments together before the day gets underway?

THE ROUTINE

1 Slow Recline: **10 reps**

2 Single Leg Lifts: **8 reps on each side**

3 Cat Cow: **10 cycles**

4 Punching Crunch: **20 reps**

Remember: Your bed is a great place to practice the seated exercises in your routines, such as the Slow Recline.

THE FUTURE: YOUR NEW DAILY HABIT

You now have a framework for building core strength as part of your everyday routine, and we hope your dedication won't stop when you put down this book. Scientists estimate it takes anywhere from 18 to 254 days for a person to form a new habit. That may seem like a long time, but it's well worth the investment.

As with forming any new habit, consistency is key. Although 5 or 10 minutes of core work every day adds up to progress, 5 minutes sporadically won't do much good. To see results, make it a daily practice. However, keep in mind that even the core can be overworked. If you experience a new pain, you may need to take a day of rest. Sore is okay; pain is not!

With long-term, daily use of your routines, you'll begin to feel your core muscles becoming stronger. When combined with nutritious food choices and some added aerobic exercise, your clothes will fit a little looser and you'll begin to see more muscle definition. Most important, you'll be lowering your risk factors for disease and decreasing the likelihood of having a fall or other injury.

You needn't rely on willpower alone to form your new habit. These tips will help you be more mindful of making core strength a daily practice.

Make a list of why you're doing it. Whatever your reasons for wanting to improve your core strength, write them down on a piece of paper and tack it up where you can see it. Being reminded of your "why" on a regular basis will help you think of your daily practice as something you *want* to do rather than something you *have* to do.

Set a reminder. If you have a smartphone, it's easy to set a daily reminder. On an iPhone, use the Clock app to set an alarm that goes off at the same time each day, or customize the time for different days of the week. There are also plenty of free apps in the App Store or Google Play Store that you can use to set up calendar notifications, text message reminders, and more. Prefer a more traditional reminder system? Use good old-fashioned sticky notes to remind you to fit in a five-minute session. Sticky notes are also great for short affirmations, such as *"I am strong,"* *"I deserve to be healthy,"* or *"I am in control of my success,"* that will help you maintain a positive mindset.

Make it part of something you enjoy. The best exercise doesn't feel like exercise at all. Make your five-minute sessions more fun by combining them with something you enjoy, such as your favorite Friday night TV show, an upbeat playlist on iTunes, or your phone calls with your grandkids.

Enlist a friend. Use the buddy system and enlist a friend to join your daily core practice, then hold each other accountable. It doesn't have to be someone you see regularly; technology such as FaceTime and Zoom makes it easier than ever to connect with friends and family even if they're on the other side of the country.

With that, we will leave you to get busy building your new, healthy habit. We applaud you for taking the first steps toward a stronger, more mobile, and more pain-free body and we wish you well on the road to self-improvement.

RESOURCES

AARP You're probably familiar with AARP, the American Association of Retired Persons. There are particularly great sections of their website focusing on healthy living and brain health, which support the strong link between your physical fitness and your longevity.

American Seniors Association ASA is an advocacy organization that lobbies for senior interests, such as preserving Medicare funding. Their website has some good resources about various benefits and programs available to seniors (e.g., insurance plans and wellness screenings).

ElderGym.com A great site for at-home fitness with resources for stretching, balance, and posture.

Fitness Over Fifty: An Exercise Guide from the National Institute on Aging This book is a favorite quick-reference material for strength, flexibility, and balance exercises. It's a great introduction for those looking to get started on a fitness program.

FitnessWithCindy.com My very own headquarters on the Internet with more than 100 free fitness videos for seniors covering cardio, strength, pain relief, and balance, along with a selection of premium fitness programs.

SeniorLifestyle.com This website covers a range of topics pertaining to independent living, such as the different options available as you age and senior-specific financial topics.

SilverSneakers.com Offered through certain Medicare plans, Silver Sneakers is a national wellness membership program for adults 65 and older. Members can use the site to access live and on-demand classes, whereas a library of articles is accessible for everyone.

National Council on Aging NCOA is all about using fact-based information to empower healthy choices. Their blog is an excellent place to learn more about senior-specific nutrition and management of chronic diseases.

Younger Next Year: The Exercise Program, by Chris Crowley and Henry S. Lodge, M.D. This is a practical but also inspirational guide to how you can use exercise to reverse the aging process.

REFERENCES

AARP. "2018 Home and Community Preferences: A National Survey of Adults Ages 18-Plus." Accessed November, 2020. AARP.org/research/topics/community/info-2018/2018-home-community-preference.html.

Centers for Disease Control and Prevention. "Keep on Your Feet—Preventing Older Adult Falls." Accessed November, 2020. CDC.gov/injury/features/older-adult-falls/index.html.

Harvard Health Publishing. "Never Too Late: Exercise Helps Late Starters." *Harvard Men's Health Watch* (blog). Accessed November, 2020. Health.Harvard.edu/mens-health/never-too-late-exercise-helps-late-starters.

Healthline. "How Long Does It Take for a New Behavior to Become Automatic?" Accessed November, 2020. Healthline.com/health/how-long-does-it-take-to-form-a-habit#tips-and-tricks.

Healthline. "Why It's Never Too Late to Start Exercising." Accessed November, 2020. Healthline.com/health-news/why-its-never-too-late-to-start-exercising.

National Council on Aging. "The 2015 United States of Aging Survey." Accessed November, 2020. https://www.unitedhealthgroup.com/content/dam/UHG/PDF/2015/USofAging-2015-Fact-Sheet.pdf.

Preidt, Robert. "Wider Waistline May Mean Shorter Lifespan: Study." *Nourish by WebMD* (blog). Accessed November, 2020. WebMD.com/diet/news/20140314/wider-waistline-may-mean-shorter-lifespan-study.

Shafrin J., Sullivan J., Goldman D. P., Gill T. M. (2017) "The association between observed mobility and quality of life in the near elderly." PLoS ONE 12(8): e0182920. https://journals.plos.org/plosone/article?id=10.1371/journal.pone.0182920.